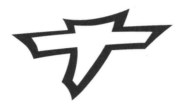

Setting Captives Free
The Lord's Table Leader's Guide

Mike Cleveland

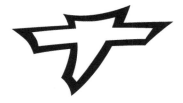

The Lord's Table
Leader's Guide

Setting Captives Free
The Lord's Table Leader's Guide
by Mike Cleveland

Inquiries should be addressed to
Focus Publishing, Rights and Permissions
PO Box 665
Bemidji, Minnesota, 56619

Scripture is taken from the
NEW AMERICAN STANDARD BIBLE,
Copyright © 1960, 1962, 1963, 1968, 1971, 1972,
1973, 1975, 1977, 1995 by the Lockman Foundation.
Used by permission.

ISBN: 1-885904-44-4

Printed in the United States of America

Introduction

The Lord's Table course is not just a diet, and it is probably unlike any other course or support group you may have encountered in the past. **The Lord's Table** places a radical emphasis on satisfying our souls in Christ. We also stress the need to repent of overeating and/or any other sinful eating habits. Though losing weight is important if we are overweight, the emphasis is on consuming Christ and developing biblical discipline in the area of eating.

If you have elected to lead a small group in this study, be encouraged to know that this Leader's Guide will give you the tools you need to be comfortable in the weeks ahead. Too often people are reluctant to be the "Leader" because they think it carries too much responsibility. You will find that with these tools and the enthusiasm of students in your group, the title of "Leader" is not intimidating at all.

Please pray at the beginning and ending of each weekly lesson. Then simply follow the lessons as printed, using care to follow the time schedule as closely as possible so that the lessons do not run long. You may decide to give the students time after the session to visit, but that should be optional. We have also included tear-out sheets you may duplicate and hand out at the end of each session to prepare students for the next week."

Strongly recommend a physical checkup with their doctors before beginning this or any other weight management program, especially if they need to adjust the eating plan for diabetes, pregnancy, or nursing moms.

In developing the Leader's Guide, we have welcomed feedback from groups who have successfully completed the course. One aspect seemed to create the most confusion, and that was the Daily Eating Schedule (page 200 in the manual). It is not mandatory that people do one lesson each day. Some people get behind while others prefer to move at a faster pace. This is fine! But working at different paces can throw off the Eating Schedule. Suggest that students copy the schedule onto a monthly calendar. They can then stay on schedule while working at a comfortable pace within the workbook.

Karen Wilkinson, Administrative Assistant at Setting Captives Free has led **The Lord's Table** group and offers the following suggestions:

I used 1 Corinthians 1:18-31 for the Scripture to encourage course participants to reject all worldly advice and all they have ever learned about dieting. God's wisdom is found in His book, and that is our only source for guidance on eating. The eating plan is a suggestion, and it is like training wheels on a bike. It is used to teach us discipline, and once we learn that, we may no longer need to follow it. We talked a little about fasting for beginners, and that it is okay to work your way up to 24 hours if necessary.
We wanted to give the students HOPE, and endeavored to do so, primarily through the testimonies which were given. We asked each course member to report their weight each week to just one person, not the whole group. Periodically, we gave the group a "total weight lost in the group" report, but did not mention amounts for any specific person.

One thing we discussed was that once they got into the course and discovered this was about much more than just our eating habits, they wanted to run away, but it was too late – sort of "once you see truth, you can't unsee it" (Steve Brown).

Karen further shares some comments from members of the course as they reached the end. You may wish to read some of these at your first session.

"...seemed as if there was a mountain ahead, but at least we had a map."
"...learned to delight in the Lord, not snacks...Psalm 37:4."
" God is big, but He is also personal."
"...favorite part was hearing about other's victories."
"...opened up a whole new world."
"...learned it's a choice between following faith or feelings."
"...discovered the selfishness of wanting to eat what, when and however she wanted."
"...gained more spiritually. God used the course to change other areas besides eating."
"...weight loss is a by-product."
"...constantly reviewing the material in the manual....life is changed!"
"...Can't thank God enough for **The Lord's Table**."

Finally, please tell your students that they may choose to join **The Lord's Table** Weekly Newsletter called 'SoulFeast' by sending a blank email to soulfeast-request@scflists.com.

Contents

Endnotes

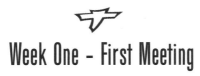

Week One - First Meeting

7:00 pm:
Begin promptly with a call to order and opening prayer.

7:05 - 7:20 pm:
Introduction of Leaders. Leaders share short testimonies related to their experience with **The Lord's Table.** These testimonies should accomplish two purposes: to honor the Lord and to give hope that change is inevitable when the principles of Scripture are followed wholeheartedly. This is a time that should immediately whet the appetite of those in attendance and provide hope that they too can be free from overeating.

7:20 - 7:30 pm:
Introduction and explanation of suggested eating plan. Care should be used to emphasize that this eating plan is not a requirement, or a diet that must be followed, but rather a "suggested eating plan" that many have followed successfully. Instruction should be given on how to eat; eat only when hungry and stop when full. There are no restrictions on the kind of food; only on how much, and worshiping the Lord with each bite.

7:30 - 7:45 pm:
Overview of the course:

    1.   Explain how to proceed through the study manual. As you introduce students to their manual, help them see that they are to begin in the "boxed" Introduction square first, then proceed to the sides of the page for additional text as well as question and answers. Explain that they can use extra sheets of paper for their answers and to keep those sheets with the manual.

    2.   Explain the principle of accountability and select accountability partners. Accountability should be daily (Hebrews 3:13), and should include the reporting of time spent with the Lord, eating habits for the day, whether or not there was exercise, and what was learned in **The Lord's Table** Bible study. It should not be a lengthy time, but can take 1-2 minutes so that it does not become a dreaded time by either partner. Accountability partners should be encouraged to decide among themselves how they will provide accountability; either through email, phone calls, fax, or in person.

3.   Introduce the schedule of the weekly group meetings. Weekly meetings should begin with opening welcome and prayer (5 minutes), proceed straight to Bible teaching (15-20 minutes), break into small groups (maximum of 12 people) to work through the questions provided (25 minutes), worship singing (5-10 minutes), and final biblical instruction and challenge (15 minutes). This will be a total of 1 hour to 1 hour and fifteen minutes. Questions for the small groups will be distributed weekly at the meetings.

7:45-7:50 pm:
Testimony of one who is experiencing victory over sin. The purpose of this testimony is to show how the application of biblical principles, combined with perseverance, produces a full heart and a disciplined body.

7:50 to 8:15 pm:
Introduction of The Lord's Table foundational teachings: The "3 D's."

Delight your soul
Discipline your body
Daily accountability

The following can be taught during the final 15-20 minutes of the first class:

Delight Your Soul: Teach from Exodus 12 (freedom begins with a "change in diet") to begin feeding on the Lamb. In Exodus 12 the Passover Lamb not only saved the Israelites from death but also provided nourishment for them. Jesus is described in Scripture as "our Passover Lamb" (1 Corinthians 5:7), "the Bread of Life" (John 6:50-58) and as "real Meat" (John 6:55). All of these food products, in the physical world, are only profitable to the body when eaten. Just so, Jesus Christ is only useful to our souls as we symbolically sink our teeth into Him; as we taste and see that He is good; as we appropriate Him into our lives. Bring in the following Scriptures:

"Your words were found, and I ate them, and Your word was to me the joy and rejoicing of my heart; for I am called by Your name" (Jeremiah 15:16).

"I have not departed from the commands of his lips; I have treasured the words of his mouth more than my daily bread" (Job 23:12).

> **"Therefore, purge out the old leaven, that you may be a new lump, since you truly are unleavened. For indeed Christ, our Passover, was sacrificed for us. Therefore let us keep the feast, not with old leaven, nor with the leaven of malice and wickedness, but with the unleavened bread of sincerity and truth" (1 Corinthians 5:7-8).**

At Jesus' birth He was immediately placed into a manger, right? But do you know what a manger is? It is that from which the animals ate. Jesus Christ was placed into a feeding trough! His birth makes a statement that He came to be fed upon. Please do not think that this teaching is "just not practical" because it doesn't contain specific calorie recommendations, foods to eat, foods to avoid...etc. Daily feeding our souls on Christ is the first step to freedom from overeating, and as time goes by we need to seek to implement this truth into our lives more and more.

The first step to being free from overeating can be summarized by the words "Delight Your Soul." In feeding on Christ the soul becomes delighted and full.

Discipline Your Body: But there are those who are truly feeding on Christ, who might even be ingesting God's Word in large amounts daily, but who do not have victory over eating habits. This is because, while they are feasting on Jesus Christ, they are not disciplining their bodies. The second principle to freedom is that we must exercise daily discipline in our eating habits. Paul says, **"But I discipline my body and bring it into subjection, lest, when I have preached to others, I myself should become disqualified" (1 Corinthians 9:27).**

Daily discipline in eating habits is why we have developed **The Lord's Table** "Eating Schedule of Normal Days, Half Days, Liquid Days and Fast Days." These are not caloric recommendations or specific food recommendations, as we do not want to focus our attention on food, but rather this combination of eating days teaches us to discipline our bodies and bring them into subjection, and to eat on purpose and with control. This way we can receive all kinds of food with thanksgiving, and we can eat in a worshipful attitude and a disciplined manner.

Remember, the second principle could be summarized by the words: "Discipline Your Body."

Daily Accountability: The third principle to freedom is accountability. Hebrews 3:13 says, **"But exhort one another daily, while it is called 'Today,' lest any of you be hardened through the deceitfulness of sin."** Daily exhortation (imploring, rebuking, encouraging) is a necessary part of avoiding sin's deception. This is the reason we have designed **The Lord's Table** local teaching and accountability groups to be interactive. Notice Ecclesiastes 4:9-12:

> **"Two are better than one, because they have a good reward for their labor. For if they fall, one will lift up his companion. But woe to him who is alone when he falls, for he has no one to help him up. Again, if two lie down together, they will keep warm; but how can one be warm alone? Though one may be overpowered by another, two can withstand him. And a threefold cord is not quickly broken."**

These verses make it clear that we cannot go it alone. We need each other. If we can find someone to walk with us daily in this goal of losing weight we will have a much better chance of succeeding.

A study was done with horses to determine the true value of team effort. The study revealed that one horse pulling alone was able to pull 2,500 pounds. The test was then repeated with two horses pulling together; the two horses were able to pull 12,500 pounds! The two horses together were able to pull 5 times the amount of weight that the one horse alone could pull! Teamwork is critical in overcoming gluttony and laziness.

Notice this thought from Matthew Henry: "Two are better than one, and more happy jointly than either of them could be separately, more pleased in one another than they could be in themselves only, mutually serviceable to each others welfare, and by a united strength more likely to do good to others."[1]

Have you ever read *Pilgrim's Progress?* It is a wonderful allegory of the Christian life. In the ninth scene a man by the name of Hope finds himself desiring to take a nap in the land of Enchantment. But young Christian reminds him of 1 Thessalonians 5:6 that says, **"let us not sleep, as do others; but let us watch and be sober."** Hope, being reminded of the truth of Scripture, becomes very thankful for Christian. He says these words: "I acknowledge that I was wrong; and if I would have been here alone, by myself sleeping I would have been in danger of death. I see it is true what that wise man said, 'Two are better than one.' Therefore you being here has been a mercy to me; and you will have a good reward for your labor."[2]

This third principle could be summarized by the words, "Daily Accountability."

The class should be closed with encouragement that persistence is the most important aspect of a successful student at **The Lord's Table.** There will come difficulties in accepting certain teachings, discouragements, struggles, victories, etc. Help the student to be forewarned that the worst thing they could do would be to quit, for then they lose both the teachings and the accountability.

The passage of Scripture that teaches this need to persevere is Luke 8:15: **"But the seed in the good soil, these are the ones who have heard the word in an honest and good heart, and hold it fast, and bear fruit with perseverance."**

The objective is not to lose 10 pounds the first two weeks. The objective is to develop habits of self-control, habits of discipline, and habits of persevering in difficult times. Some will want to become extreme and cut calories way down. This is counterproductive for the less calories consumed, the slower the metabolism functions and the less fat the body burns. Normal eating when hungry and stopping when full, utilizing small portions of food, combined with daily exercise of some kind (any kind) is the most effective way to lose weight. Encourage the student that perseverance is half of the battle and that those who persevere will "bear fruit" in self-control and discipline.

Note: Following is a Handout Sheet you may copy to send home with members of the class. These questions will be answered in next week's lesson.

Handout Questions for Group Discussion
Week 2

Day 1
Question 1. According to 1 Corinthians 10:31, what actions are included in those which should be done for God's glory? When this verse sinks into your soul, what does the Holy Spirit say to you? Specifically, how will this truth affect your life, your eating habits, etc.?

Question 2. What aspects of God's character are mentioned in Psalm 115:1 as reasons for giving glory to His name? What is mercy? What is truth?

Question 3. Instead of filling ourselves with food, how do we, instead, become filled with hope? (Romans 15:13).

Day 2
Question 4. Where do we find true nourishment for our souls? (John 6:53:58).

Question 5. Isaiah 55:2 says, "**Listen carefully to Me, and eat what is good**." In effect, God is saying here that the richest food is eaten with our ears. What does this mean?

Question 6. What does fullness in Christ mean to you? (Colossians 2:9-10).

Day 3
Question 7. From Psalm 81:10-12, what two principles will provide victory over habitual sin?

Question 8. According to Jeremiah 15:16, what does it mean to eat God's Word? How do we develop an appetite for God's Word so that it becomes our joy and delight?

Day 4
Question 9. What is our reward if our purpose in fasting is to be noticed by others? Who rewards us when we fast without fanfare? (Matthew 6:16).

Day 5

Question 10. According to Colossians 2:20-23, what is the problem with the teaching of the diet craze industry today?

Question 11. According to 1 Corinthians 1:19-20, 25, what should we trust in for a solution to our food issues?

Question 12. According to 1 Timothy 4:1-5 who is able to receive all food with thanksgiving? (Those who believe and know the truth). These verses give us a warning and a hope. How do they apply to our eating?

Week Two

7:00-7:05:
Call to Order and Opening Prayer

7:05-7:25:
Teaching: Success! (Psalm 1– see below).

7:25-7:30:
Small break and reorganize into small groups

7:30-7:55:
Small Group Interaction

7:55-8:05:
Coming back together, singing two to three songs.

8:05-8:15:
Teaching and Challenge: Victory Through Repentance (Acts 26:16-18).

Teaching: Success!

[1]How blessed is the man who does not walk in the counsel of the wicked, nor stand in the path of sinners, nor sit in the seat of scoffers! [2]But his delight is in the law of the LORD, and in His law he meditates day and night. [3]He will be like a tree firmly planted by streams of water, which yields its fruit in its season and its leaf does not wither; and in whatever he does, he prospers. [4]The wicked are not so, but they are like chaff which the wind drives away. [5]Therefore the wicked will not stand in the judgment, nor sinners in the assembly of the righteous. [6]For the LORD knows the way of the righteous, but the way of the wicked will perish (Psalm 1:1-6).

Helps for teachers:
This passage promises a successful Christian walk if the truths it conveys are followed. These truths refer both to the actions (v. 1) and the heart (v. 2). The qualities that bring success in the Christian life are:

- Refusing to follow (actions) the counsel of the wicked, nor to walk in the paths of sinners or to sit with mockers. Help the class to understand the reality that worldly counsel is detrimental to our walk in the Lord, and in the area of dieting worldly counselors abound.
- Delighting in (heart) God's Word and God's ways. Not only do we avoid the errors of the world and the life of the ungodly, but we seek to delight in the Lord. Our hearts must become involved in the seeking of and enjoyment of the Lord. This enjoyment of God comes from following the Lord, from walking in and obeying His commands.

The promise for avoiding worldly counsel and sinful ways, and for delighting in God's Word, is success (v. 3). For our study, help the class to see that their "success" in losing weight will be in direct proportion to their avoidance of worldly input in dieting, and of their embracing of and drinking in the Truth of God's Word.

A tree only produces fruit when it drinks in the nutrients of the available water. In the same way, the fruitfulness of weight loss comes by drinking in the Truth of God's Word and living it out. Encourage the class to begin living by the streams of water in God's Word, to drink of them often, to begin living what they are learning. Challenge them to begin turning to God and His Word for all the stresses they face in life, for all the trials that God will bring, for any loneliness and boredom they endure. Help them to form habits of automatically turning to the Lord, of opening His Word, of seeking His face, in times of difficulty and stress.

Verse 4 presents the emptiness of the wicked. It compares them to chaff, that empty shell that has no life in it. This emptiness is one thing that propels the "addiction" of those who turn to drugs, alcohol, or food for fullness. True fullness can only be found in Jesus and in having a relationship with Him. Encourage the class to examine if they have "fullness of joy in believing" (Romans 15:13) or whether they are empty, like chaff.

Verses 5 and 6 present a promise and a warning having to do with the "way" of the godly and the "way" of the wicked. God watches over the way of the godly but the way of the wicked will perish. The class needs to understand that the kingdom of God is not about words but rather about power to live a different life (1 Corinthians 4:20). It is the way of men and women that is discussed in Psalm 1, not their words. The life lived shouts louder than the words spoken. Man can fool man with words, but God sees man's "ways."

This first teaching session should be ended with this challenge: Do you want to profit in all you do? Do you want to be successful in losing weight? Then begin to turn your back on worldly counselors and methods, and sinful ways of living, and instead learn how to delight your heart in the Lord by following Him, His Word, and His ways.

Day 1

Question 1. According to 1 Corinthians 10:31, what actions are included in those which should be done for God's glory? When this verse sinks into your soul, what does the Holy Spirit say to you? Specifically, how will this truth affect your life, your eating habits, etc.?

> The biblical motive for weight loss is the glory of God: **"Whether, then, you eat or drink or whatever you do, do all to the glory of God" (1 Corinthians 10:31)**. This means that the motivation of our hearts must be to glorify God with our eating, with our exercise, with our entire lives. Help the students to understand that God's glory is the only motive which will stand the test of time, and that disciplined eating and daily exercise is honoring to God.
>
> Sometimes people rush right into a meal without considering how they may honor the Lord in that particular meal. Sometimes they do not see that their eating and drinking is to be done for God's glory. Encourage students to slow down and to worship God with every bite they take, and to make sure that God is honored with the amount they eat.

On the answer to this question, allow the students to express how they will apply the truth in their own lives. Answers should be that the student will begin, by the Holy Spirit, to consciously eat to the glory of God and to consciously exercise in some manner every day. The answers should state that the student has seen how in the past they have had wrong motives, and how they see that true motivation is important in losing weight, as well as in all of life.

Question 2. What aspects of God's character are mentioned in Psalm 115:1 as reasons for giving glory to His name? What is mercy? What is truth? **"Not to us, O LORD, not to us, but to Your name give glory because of Your lovingkindness, because of Your truth" (Psalm 115:1).**

God is deserving of glory because of His grace, because of His love, because of His truth, because of all His character traits. This is a good point to help the students to focus upon the character of God, His unchanging nature, His attributes. Help them to see that He is "altogether lovely" and that because of the beauty of His character He is worthy of glory. Help them to see that **The Lord's Table** course seeks to provide focused attention upon God because it is as we view God that we become changed into His image:

"But whenever a person turns to the Lord, the veil is taken away. Now the Lord is the Spirit, and where the Spirit of the Lord is, there is liberty. But we all, with unveiled face, beholding as in a mirror the glory of the Lord, are being transformed into the same image from glory to glory, just as from the Lord, the Spirit" (2 Corinthians 3:17-18).

It is just at this point that the world fails in truly assisting men and women to freedom from overeating. The focus of the worldly counselors is on food, not on Christ. Yet it is as we turn to the Lord and view His glory (the beauty of His character and attributes), as revealed in His Son, that we are "transformed into the same image." This transformation is what we are after here at **The Lord's Table**, therefore we must constantly seek to point men and women to the Lord and call them to turn to Him.

Psalm 115:1 says that God is deserving of glory because of His attributes of grace and truth. These attributes are most clearly revealed in Jesus Christ, Who is "full of grace and truth" (John 1:14).

Question 3. Instead of filling ourselves with food, how do we, instead, become filled with hope? **"Now may the God of hope fill you with all joy and peace in believing, so that you will abound in hope by the power of the Holy Spirit" (Romans 15:13).**

There is a fullness of joy and fullness of peace to be found in believing God. This fullness of soul is a preventative to the emptiness that can lead to overeating and should be taught to the students as that which is the alternative to overeating. Simply sitting down with a passage of God's Word and purposefully believing it's every verse, with the desire to act upon it, brings fullness of delight.

Day 2

Question 4. Where do we find true nourishment for our souls? (John 6:53:58).

> True nourishment for our souls is found in Jesus Christ as He is presented to us as "True Food" (verse 53) and the "Bread of Life" (verse 58).

Question 5. Isaiah 55:2 says, **"Listen carefully to Me, and eat what is good."** In effect, God is saying here that the richest food is eaten with our ears. What does this mean?

> When we listen to God's Word we are feeding on spiritual food. 1 Timothy 4:6 should be brought in here to affirm the truth that God's Word is nourishment to the soul. In reality, when we "eat with our ears," praise comes out of our mouths instead of food going in.

Question 6. What does fullness in Christ mean to you? (Colossians 2:9-10).

> There is no right or wrong answer here; simply allow the students to think through this passage and formulate their own answers.

Day 3

Question 7. From Psalm 81:10-12, what two principles will provide victory over habitual sin?

> The two principles stated in Psalm 81:10-12 are:
>   1. Eagerly Feeding on God's Word (verse 10)
>   2. Obedience (verse 11)

Question 8. According to Jeremiah 15:16 what does it mean to eat God's Word? How do we develop an appetite for God's Word so that it becomes our joy and delight?

> This question does not necessarily have a right/wrong answer; rather it is to stimulate discussion and get input from the students. The idea is to convey that there is real nourishment in God's Word if it is read and obeyed, and the results of feeding on His Word brings fullness to the soul and delight to the heart.

Day 4

Question 9. What is our reward if our purpose in fasting is to be noticed by others? Who rewards us when we fast without fanfare? (Matthew 6:16-18).

> If we fast with wrong motives, such as to appear spiritual or in some other way call attention to ourselves, the reward we have is the attention of others. Whereas if we fast in secret, that is, without calling attention to ourselves, God Himself rewards us.
>
> It is important for the students to understand about fasting. This would be a good time to highly recommend the book called *A Hunger for God* by John Piper.[3]

Day 5

Question 10. According to Colossians 2:20-23, what is the problem with the teaching of the diet craze industry today?

> The diet industry instructs us to "taste not, touch not" some type of food. There is an appearance of wisdom in this denial of certain foods, yet it contains no power to restrain our flesh. We are overweight not because we happen to eat the wrong kinds of foods, or that we have been combining foods in the wrong way, the problem is that we are prone to indulge our flesh. This legalistic restricting of certain foods does not provide the liberty Christians have in the gospel.

Question 11. According to 1 Corinthians 1:19-20, 25, what should we trust in for a solution to our food issues?

> 1 Corinthians 1:19-20, 25 show us the supreme value of having God's wisdom for living, and contrasts that wisdom with the wisdom of man. The wisdom of man is said to be foolishness in comparison to God's wisdom. Help the students to understand that it truly is foolishness to follow man's "wisdom" when it comes to finding freedom from sinful habits.

Question 12. According to 1 Timothy 4:1-5 who is able to receive all food with thanksgiving? These verses give us a warning and a hope. How do they apply to our eating?

> 1 Timothy 4:1-5 tell us that those who believe and know the truth (verse 3) are able to receive all food with thanksgiving. The warning given is to not pay attention to those who teach the religion of denial of God-given gifts, such as marriage and food. The hope is that if we know this truth we can "reject nothing" (verse 4) and "gratefully share" in all things God gives us. In other words, we can be free from the control of food as we realize that we don't have to focus on denying certain foods, or how to combine foods the right way, or how many calories, carbs or fat grams are in a particular food.

Warning: This particular area of teaching is controversial, and in a large crowd there may be some who, because of indoctrination from the diet craze industry, or because of teachings by legalistic religions, state strongly that certain foods are to be avoided. They may go so far as to dogmatically state that no individual or program could possibly be "Christian" if it doesn't teach the denial of certain meats, sugars, etc... They may point to Old Testament prohibitions against eating certain meat, or to "scientific" studies that show certain foods are hazard to our health.

It is important that class time not be taken up in argument on this issue. The teacher may need to state strongly that the subject can be discussed after class, and to simply move on. It is also important for the teacher to "believe and know the truth" that all foods are to be received with thanksgiving, and to be well acquainted with the following passages of Scripture:

> Mark 7:14-23
> Acts 10:9-15

Romans 14:14-22
Colossians 2:20-23
1 Timothy 4:1-5

8:05-8:15 pm:
Final Teaching and Challenge: Victory Through Repentance

**"But get up and stand on your feet; for this purpose I have appeared
to you, to appoint you a minister and a witness not only to the things
which you have seen, but also to the things in which I will appear to
you; rescuing you from the Jewish people and from the Gentiles, to
whom I am sending you, to open their eyes so that they may turn from
darkness to light and from the dominion of Satan to God, that they may
receive forgiveness of sins and an inheritance among those who have
been sanctified by faith in Me" (Acts 26:16-18).**

Helps for teachers:
This passage defines the word "repentance." Repentance is not simply
turning away from sin, it is both turning away from sin and turning to God.
Paul was going to be used by God to turn men and women away from
darkness and to the light, away from the dominion of Satan and to God.
So repentance is what breaks the power of sin because I turn from slavery
to sin and become enslaved to the power of God instead. It is only when
we become captives to Christ in reality that we are free from captivity to
overeating.

"Darkness" in Scripture refers to error, deception, secrecy, bondage, sin. For
our purposes, help the class to see that repentance is when I turn away from
any hiding of food, or eating in secret, or deception in my accountability
reports, or bondage to overeating when stressed, tired, lonely or bored.
When I turn to the "light" I begin living a life that is transparent and open,
that can be seen by all. It is a pure life, it is a life of no hiding, no deception,
no darkness of habitual sin.

The reason we want to discuss the issue of repentance is because in the
coming week the course teaches about repentance, and there is a need to
prepare the students' hearts and minds for what happens in repentance. The
student may be surprised by sin. When we ask God to show us what is in

our hearts, He will do it–and it is not a pretty picture. The heart is deceitful above all things, who can know it? This should not be discouraging to the student, rather they should recognize this is God's way of bringing hidden sin out into the light. Once they see it, they can repent of it and go on.

It would be good to "pre-warn" the class of this "shock" of seeing sin in the heart by encouraging the class to read what Sue Bohlin, speaker and webservant for Probe Ministries has written regarding the changes that happen in repentance found on Day 7 of **The Lords Table** manual. This will be discussed at the next lesson.

At **The Lord's Table** we call overeating sin, and the solution is repentance. There is a reason for this as said by John Alexander:

"Sin is the best news there is, the best news there could be in our predicament. Because with sin, there's a way out. There's the possibility of repentance. You can't repent of confusion or psychological flaws inflicted by your parents–you're stuck with them. But you can repent of sin. Sin and repentance are the only grounds for hope and joy."

> John Alexander in *The Other Side*
> (Christianity Today, Vol. 39, no. 1, Jan-Feb, 1993).

The devil presents repentance as a fatal day, the day when my heart dies because I must give up what it loves. But the devil lies, for repentance is not a fatal day but rather a natal day, a day when new life begins and new love emerges in my heart to replace the old.

Finally, by way of closing the meeting, simply issue a challenge to make sure that in the coming weeks they are evidencing genuine repentance in all areas; not just in eating, but in any other area in which there is sin in their life.

Handout the Question sheet for the next meeting. Close in prayer.

Handout Questions for Group Discussion
Week 3

Day 6

Question 1. According to John 6:29, what work does God require of us?

Question 2. What is the promised result of taking in God's Word, and how does this apply to us? (Isaiah 55:10-11).

Question 3. What biblical teaching in **The Lord's Table** makes it different from secular weight loss programs?

Day 7

Question 4. What does it mean to be poor in spirit? How do we know if humility and spiritual poverty are present in our lives? (Matthew 5:1-3).

Question 5. What reward is given to the poor in spirit? (Matthew 5:3).

Question 6. Why is it important that we come to Christ with spiritual poverty?

Day 8

Question 7. According to 1 Peter 2:21-25, why did Jesus die for our sins?

Question 8. What is the source of our power to overcome the sin of overeating? (1 Corinthians 1:18).

Day 9

Question 9. What does it mean to hunger and thirst for righteousness? What is the result? (Matthew 5:6).

Day 10

Question 10. What contrast is mentioned in Isaiah 55:1-3? For this particular study on weight loss, how do these contrasts apply to us?

Week Three

7:00-7:05:
Call to Order and Opening Prayer

7:05-7:25:
Teaching: Looking to Jesus (Hebrews 12:1-4 below).
Prepare and read this before class time.

7:25-7:30:
Small break and reorganize into small groups

7:30-7:55:
Small Group Interaction

7:55-8:05:
Coming back together, singing two to three songs

8:05-8:15:
Teaching and Challenge: Delighting in Jesus (Psalm 37:4-5).

Looking to Jesus

[1]"Therefore, since we have so great a cloud of witnesses surrounding us, let us also lay aside every encumbrance and the sin which so easily entangles us, and let us run with endurance the race that is set before us, [2]fixing our eyes on Jesus, the author and perfecter of faith, who for the joy set before Him endured the cross, despising the shame, and has sat down at the right hand of the throne of God. [3]For consider Him who has endured such hostility by sinners against Himself, so that you will not grow weary and lose heart. [4]You have not yet resisted to the point of shedding blood in your striving against sin" (Hebrews 12:1-4).

Helps for teachers:
This passage exhorts us to run our race with endurance, and teaches us how to run: by looking at Jesus. There is tremendous value in fixing our eyes on Jesus, for more is accomplished against sin by looking to Jesus than by all the self-effort we could ever muster. While the world focuses on food;

calories, points, fat grams and carbs; the Bible turns us to Jesus Christ, and as we look at Jesus we are transformed into His image. Yes, at **The Lord's Table**, we are on the "Jesus Watchers" program, and the results are dramatic!

The word "fixing" in verse two has to do with avoiding that which would distract so as to look intently at Jesus. The word "consider" in verse three has to do with purposeful thinking and meditation. So we are to avoid that which would distract us from looking at Jesus and we are to purposely think about and meditate on Him.

Verse 1 tells us that we are to rid our lives of anything that hinders our running the race of life, and especially to lay aside the thornlike sin that entangles and causes us to stumble..

Verses 2 and 3 tell us that focusing on Christ will enable us to endure and not become discouraged. Help the class understand that in losing weight there is a cross of pain to endure, and the way to keep from losing heart is to look to Jesus. Help them apply this passage to their struggle against sin, and to show them Jesus Who endured the cross and was victorious. Help them to see from verse 3 that we can either become discouraged and lose heart, or we can look to Jesus, but we cannot do both at the same time. This is one of the tremendous benefits that comes to the Christian, that by focusing on Jesus we are given supernatural strength to press on.

During the study last week, the class focused on repentance. Now we are encouraging the radical focus of attention upon Jesus Christ. This is a logical flow in sequence for repentance includes turning away from focusing on food and turning our attention instead to Jesus. We are to be just as focused on Christ as we once were on food. This is what it looks like for those involved in gluttony to repent.

It's not that we are to begin thinking that food is bad; it's that we simply change focus from food to Christ. We can still enjoy our food, and even more so because we will learn to worship God with each bite, but we find that our passion is no longer food but Jesus Christ. We redirect our interest, our attention, our passion, our desires to Jesus and away from food. This is fixing our eyes on Jesus, not allowing any distractions, and purposefully thinking about and concentrating on Him.

Day 6

Question 1. According to John 6:29, what work does God require of us?

> According to Jesus in John 6:29 the "works of God" are that we believe in Jesus. To apply this teaching to our study on weight loss, it is important for the student to understand that they should not be pursuing weight loss as a "work" to gain God's favor. The works that God requires is belief in His Son.

Question 2. What is the promised result of taking in God's Word, and how does this apply to us? (Isaiah 55:10-11).

> The Word of God produces fruit. One of the 'fruits' that we desire in our lives is 'self control" and the ability to turn from self-indulgence. This comes as a direct result of the application of biblical principles in our lives. **"Sanctify them in the truth; Your word is truth" (John 17:17).**

Question 3. What biblical teaching in **The Lord's Table** makes it different from secular weight loss programs?

> Quote from **The Lord's Table Manual** (page 17): "This teaching is the essence of what makes **The Lord's Table** different from secular weight management programs, and the understanding and implementation of this truth will mean your victory over old eating habits. We are simply stating here that Christ is real food for the soul, and to embrace Him and feed on Him produces freedom from life dominating and/or habitual sin."

Day 7

Question 4. What does it mean to be poor in spirit? How do we know if humility and spiritual poverty are present in our lives? (Matthew 5:1-3).

> Poverty of spirit is recognition that I am nothing and I have nothing apart from Christ. It is to declare myself spiritually bankrupt outside of Christ. It is a full recognition and confession of my bondage to sin apart from God's grace.

We can tell when God has worked this poverty of spirit in us when we become desperate for Him, when we seek Him with our whole hearts, when we forsake our sin and begin to cling to Christ.

This poverty of spirit is the opposite of those who come to Him reciting their good deeds, or their spiritual conquests, or their supposedly good character traits.

Question 5. What reward is given to the poor in spirit? (Matthew 5:3).

The reward given to the poor in spirit is "the kingdom of heaven." We go from paupers to princes when we come to Christ empty handed. The kingdom of heaven is not given to those who are full of the kingdom of this world, but rather to those who have been emptied of self, and to those who are through with sin.

Don't allow the students to go off on a "rabbit trail" on the definition here of "kingdom of heaven" (salvation in Christ), but rather keep the focus on what it means to be spiritually impoverished and then graciously enriched in Christ.

Question 6. Why is it important that we come to Christ with spiritual poverty?

Jesus does not fill hands that are already full. In order to experience the blessing of the grace of God we must become broken and empty before Him. He fills and enriches those who admit their spiritual bankruptcy apart from Christ. Applying this to weight loss, help the students to understand that it is only as we come to Jesus helpless, admitting our weakness and inability to overcome the lusts of the flesh, that He will energize us by grace and live His victory through us. Those who come to Him with something to offer, or as well-educated teachers, holding to their own understanding, etc. will need to experience this spiritual poverty before they will experience God's assistance.

Day 8

Question 7. According to 1 Peter 2:21-25, why did Jesus die for our sins?

Jesus died for our sins, "so that we might die to sin and live to righteousness." It is important that we understand that one of the reasons Jesus died on the cross was to accomplish our death to sin. He died for us that we might live for righteousness. Help the students apply this teaching by encouraging them to understand that one of the reasons Jesus died for our sins was that we might die to overeating. He died for us that we might live in self-control, overcoming our flesh, and walking in victory by His grace.

Question 8. What is the source of our power to overcome the sin of overeating? (1 Corinthians 1:18).

According to 1 Corinthians 1:18, the cross is the power of God for us who are being saved. Focusing on the cross will reveal to us that our sins are forgiven and that our old nature is crucified with Christ. Looking at the cross shows us that Jesus suffered to remove our guilt and shame, and that He died for us that we might live for Him. The cross is not just the doorway to heaven; it is also the pathway to daily victory over the flesh.

Day 9

Question 9. What does it mean to hunger and thirst for righteousness? What is the result? (Matthew 5:6).

Hungering and thirsting for righteousness is that state of eagerly craving righteousness. Like a thirsty man in the desert searching for water, those who thirst for righteousness are singularly focused on acquiring that which they need. There is a very real sense that we must have righteousness or we will perish.

The result of this hungering and thirsting for righteousness is that we are filled with righteousness, literally that we become filled with God. Help the students understand that the purpose of **The Lord's Table** Bible study is to create a hunger within them that leads to a fullness of Jesus Christ.

Day 10

Question 10. What contrast is mentioned in Isaiah 55:1-3? For this particular study on weight loss, how do these contrasts apply to us?

> The contrast presented in Isaiah 55:1-3 is that of spending time and money on what does not satisfy and ending up empty, versus listening carefully to God and delighting in abundance.
>
> It is important for the students to understand that in overeating we are spending ourselves on that which does not satisfy, and to assist them in changing from overeating food to listening carefully to God's Word.

8:05-8:15 pm:
Final Teaching and Challenge: Delighting in Jesus

"Delight yourself in the LORD; And He will give you the desires of your heart. Commit your way to the LORD, Trust also in Him, and He will do it" (Psalm 37:4-5).

Helps for teachers:
These verses of Scripture will no doubt change the view that many people have of God. The verses show us that God is a God who wants His children to delight in Him. In fact, He desires us to delight in Him so much that when we do, He gives us the desires of our heart.

There are three specific things that must be true in order to delight in God:

> 1. We must know God. This is the personal relationship we have with God in salvation, as He turns our hearts away from sin and turns us to His Son. **"This is eternal life, that they may know You, the only true God, and Jesus Christ whom You have sent" (John 17:3).** We are unable to delight in someone whom we do not know.
>
> 2. We must know that God is at work to do us good in all things. Yes, we must believe that **"God causes all things to work together for good to those who love God, to those who are called according to His purpose" (Romans 8:28).** Otherwise our circumstances could remove our delight in God.

26

3. We must have assurance of future and eternal pleasure in Christ. Otherwise our delight would be temporary. **"You will make known to me the path of life; in Your presence is fullness of joy; in Your right hand there are pleasures forever" (Psalm 16:11).**

This is an excellent time to help the class see that the greatest desire of God for His children is that they would find their greatest delight in Him. Help them to understand that in the past we have found our greatest delight in food, rather than in God, and that was truly idolatry. We are not to find our supreme delight in food, or in anything created, but rather in God the Creator, Redeemer and Sustainer of all.

The promise for those who delight in the Lord is that they would receive the desires of their heart. But this promise is far more than a heavenly slot-machine where we put in delight in God and out pops a new car. No, as we delight in the Lord He Himself becomes the desire of our hearts. As we delight in Him He gives us more enjoyment in Him as a reward.

Someone has once said that our souls are worth what our hearts delight in. Challenge the class, as they prepare to leave, to examine what their hearts truly delight in, and help them to see that God is to be our greatest Delight, and that we gain the desires of our heart as we delight in Him. Losing weight can be granted to us by God as we seek Him first and delight in Him most.

Hand out the question sheets for next week's lesson. Close in prayer.

Handout Questions for Group Discussion
Week 4

Day 11
Question 1. In repentance, why is it necessary to do a complete 180 degree turn?

Question 2. According to 2 Timothy 2:25-26, what is God's part in repentance? What is our part? What are the results of repentance?

Day 12
Question 3. What is the biblical term for overeating?

Question 4. What is the purpose of calling overeating sin? (repentance, sweet refreshment).

Day 13
Question 5. What is the key to lasting victory over sin?

Question 6. What is the relationship between repentance & worship?

Day 14
Question 7. Why is it absolutely necessary to experience a total change in our appetite?

Question 8. Read Romans 13:14. What does it mean to put on Christ? In what practical ways can we stop making provision for overeating?

Day 15
Question 9. According to Hebrews 3:13, why do we need accountability?

Question 10. What are some ways we can encourage each other in this battle as we are instructed in Hebrews 10:23-25?

Week Four

7:00-7:05:
Call to Order and Opening Prayer

7:05-7:25:
Teaching: Worship (Revelation 4:8-11, below).

7:25-7:30:
Small break and reorganize into small groups

7:30-7:55:
Small Group Interaction

7:55-8:05:
Coming back together, singing two to three songs

8:05-8:15:
Teaching and Challenge: Worship Illustrated (Luke 7:37-39; 47-49).

Worship

[8]And the four living creatures, each one of them having six wings, are full of eyes around and within; and day and night they do not cease to say, "HOLY, HOLY, HOLY is THE LORD GOD, THE ALMIGHTY, WHO WAS AND WHO IS AND WHO IS TO COME." [9]And when the living creatures give glory and honor and thanks to Him who sits on the throne, to Him who lives forever and ever, [10]the twenty-four elders will fall down before Him who sits on the throne, and will worship Him who lives forever and ever, and will cast their crowns before the throne, saying, [11]"Worthy are You, our Lord and our God, to receive glory and honor and power; for You created all things, and because of Your will they existed, and were created" (Revelation 4:8-11).

Helps for teachers:
This passage in Revelation 4 speaks to us about how worship is done in heaven. We want the students to view this heavenly worship experience

right at the beginning of class today, and to somehow enter in to the enjoyment of that worship right along with those in heaven. Let's look at the characteristics of true worship, and challenge ourselves and our students to carry this kind of worship with us throughout our days.

First, this passage makes it clear that true worship is God-centered. The worship creatures extol the praise of "The Lord God," "the Almighty," (verse 8) to "Him who sits on the throne" and "who lives forever and ever" (verse 9), and they worship "our Lord and our God" who created all things. True worship is first and foremost consumed with God. This is opposite of those who live in this world with every thought being for themselves, or even of true Christians, who being immature are yet focused on self. Our world revolves correctly when we are no longer at the center, when God has dethroned self and has taken His rightful position in our lives as Lord, King, Master and Ruler, and when our hearts are consumed with Him.

Second, this passage teaches us that true worship is reciting the worth of God. The creatures in heaven declare, "Worthy are you, our Lord and our God" (verse 11). The great unnumbered multitude in Revelation 5 also declares the worth of God and of the Lamb:

[11] Then I looked, and I heard the voice of many angels around the throne and the living creatures and the elders; and the number of them was myriads of myriads, and thousands of thousands, [12] saying with a loud voice, "Worthy is the Lamb that was slain to receive power and riches and wisdom and might and honor and glory and blessing." [13] And every created thing which is in heaven and on the earth and under the earth and on the sea, and all things in them, I heard saying, "To Him who sits on the throne, and to the Lamb, be blessing and honor and glory and dominion forever and ever" (Revelation 5:11-13).

Third, true worship of God is accomplished by a life of submission to God. The elders "fall down before Him" and worship Him in the posture of submission. Those who bow the knee to God, living a life of submission to Him, are master of their cravings. Because they fall down before God they can stand tall against temptation, and through worship of God they are free from idolatry.

Fourth, this passage makes it clear that this worship is continual; "night and day they do not cease" (verse 8). Real worship of God should not take just take place in church on Sundays, but is to be a 24/7/365 experience for the believer. We are to worship God "night and day." One of the greatest times of worship can be experienced while eating. If we will slow down and purposefully concentrate on the Lord as we take each bite, we will worship Him in spirit and in truth through a whole meal. With each bite we can extol the beauty and virtues of our God: Bite 1, He is Holy; Bite 2, He is Just; Bite 3, He is Gracious, Bite 4, He is the Creator of all things; Bite 5, He is the Lamb of God who takes away the sin of the world; Bite 6, He is the Savior of all who repent and believe; Bite 7, He is the Friend of sinners, etc...

Finally, this teaching is not at all disconnected from weight loss. The one who takes this teaching to heart and turns from a self-pleasing and flesh-gratifying life, to a life centered in God, who learns to extol the worth of God continually, who lives in submission to God, who enjoys meals now because they are an experience of deep worship, will inevitably lose weight. Our focus is no longer on food, but on God. Our hearts are taken up with God. As we turn our eyes upon Him the things of earth grow strangely dim, in the light of His glory and grace.

At this point the teacher can challenge the class to begin living a life of true worship of God, making a complete turn away from overeating and laziness. Our lives are to be God-centered, extolling the virtues of our Great God and Savior, and to be doing this continually, night and day. Those who are saved from a life of sin find it quite easy to worship God continually, and this worship of God should include every area of our lives, including our times of eating.

Conclude this time of teaching and worship with this excellent poem:

Worship the Lamb
William Claire Greiner

Come with singing unto Zion,
Enter through the gates with praise;
In the royal courts of splendor,
Tell of Love's redeeming grace;
Let God's majesty enfold you,
While the angels "Holy!" cry;
Worship at the throne of mercy,
Christ the Lamb to glorify.

Blood-bought souls of ev'ry nation
Stand united at the throne;
All their thoughts and their devotion
Are for One and One alone;
Glory, honor, power and blessing,
Lamb of God we give to Thee;
Young and old Thy name confessing,
In glad homage bend the knee.

Precious Savior, we adore Thee,
Be exalted here to today;
May Thy name be highly honored
In the things we do and say;
With the saints of all the ages,
At Thy feet we prostrate fall,
We enthrone Thee with our worship,
And proclaim Thee Lord of all!

Come and worship the Lamb!
Worship the Lamb!
At His feet let us worship the Lamb!
Royal diadem bring;
Christ is Lord! Crown Him King!
Oh, come and worship the Lamb!

William Claire Greiner
1989, Used by Permission

Day 11

Question 1. In repentance, why is it necessary to do a complete 180 degree turn?

Repentance is a complete "about face" turn away from sin, and turn to God. The importance of this full turn cannot be overemphasized.

If we were to just turn away from sin, but didn't make a complete turn to Christ, we would be open and exposed to either returning to the same sin or simply replacing one sin with another. Our hearts are designed to be captive, and they will either find that captivity in sin or in Jesus. In repentance we go from being sin-slaves to being Son-slaves, and both are important. Paul was once enslaved to sin but through repentance he had become "enslaved to God" (Romans 6:22). Part of Jesus' work was to "take captivity captive" (Ephesians 4:8) so that those who were formerly captive to the power of sin and to the influence of the devil now become captives of Christ and to the freedom of the gospel.

This is an excellent place to help the students see that we at **The Lord's Table** are not just about losing weight, but rather we are about helping hearts become captive to Christ.

Question 2. According to 2 Timothy 2:25-26, what is God's part in repentance? What is our part? What are the results of repentance?

According to 2 Timothy 2:25-26, it is God alone who grants repentance to sinners. This is important to understand, for only as we understand that it is God's work to turn people from sin and place them in His Son, can we exercise the "patience" that is called for in this passage. We are looking for the students to grasp the concept that repentance is a gift, given by our Sovereign God, to those whom He chooses.

A warning needs to be given here. We cannot say "if A, then B" with this particular teaching. Some will attempt to disagree with this teaching that God grants repentance stating, "Well, if that is true, then we don't need to witness to or pray for people, because God will grant repentance to whomever He wishes." No, this statement is not true, for we are commanded by God to witness to every creature and to pray for all men. We cannot say "if A, then B" for it is entirely possible that A could be true but not B as in this case. (Please be familiar with Appendix A before teaching this session).

Day 12

Question 3. What is the biblical term for overeating?

The biblical term for overeating is "gluttony."

Question 4. What is the purpose of calling overeating sin?

The purpose of truthful speaking regarding overeating is that blessings only come to those who repent. We cannot repent of a low metabolism, we cannot repent of a genetic disorder, we can only repent of sin. And when we turn away from sin and begin seeking the Lord, we experience the "times of refreshing" that are promised in Scripture to those who repent (see Acts 3:19).

We are definitely not teaching that we ignore physical problems. We acknowledge that there are physical problems that require the expertise of the medical profession. We are saying that we need to acknowledge habitual overeating as sin, as gluttony, and accept the biblical solution of repentance, rather than make excuses which will only keep us in bondage.

Day 13

Question 5. What is the key to lasting victory over sin?

Repentance is the key to lasting victory over sin. This is important to understand, for repentance is that which sends us in a different direction; it turns us away from indulging our flesh and making excuses, it turns us from deception and sinful bondage.

Question 6. What is the relationship between repentance and worship?

Repentance and worship go hand in hand, as repentance leads to true worship of God. The repentant person becomes consumed with God, even as they were previously consumed with sin. Ecclesiastes 5:1-2, 7 shows us how repentance and worship go together, and how "awe" of God comes from a repentant heart.

Day 14

Question 7. Why is it absolutely necessary to experience a total change in our appetite?

> People who lose weight but do not feed on Christ could eventually end up being worse off than they were before they lost the weight. The reason is because "nature abhors a vacuum," which is just another way of saying that we were designed to worship something. If we cease worshiping food, but don't have our appetite for worship satisfied in Christ, then we will search elsewhere for something to worship and could get into a much worse condition. Please study Luke 11:24-26 in preparation for this day's teaching.

Question 8. What does it mean to put on Christ? (Romans 13:14). In what practical ways can we stop making provision for overeating?

> No right or wrong answers here, just encourage class discussion and input.

Day 15

Question 9. According to Hebrews 3:13, why do we need accountability?

> According to Hebrews 3:13, daily encouragement and accountability is a preventative to hardening of the heart through the deceitfulness of sin.

Question 10. What are some ways we can encourage each other in this battle as we are instructed in Hebrews 10:23-25?

> There are no right and wrong answers to this question. Encourage student input as to the ways they encourage one another daily, so that the class may profit from discussing this truth.

8:05-8:15 pm:
Final Teaching and Challenge: Worship Illustrated

And there was a woman in the city who was a sinner; and when she learned that He (Jesus) was reclining at the table in the Pharisee's house, she brought an alabaster vial of perfume, and standing behind Him at His feet, weeping, she began to wet His feet with her tears, and kept wiping them with the hair of her head, and kissing His feet and anointing them with the perfume. Now when the Pharisee who had invited Him saw this, he said to himself, "If this man were a prophet He would know who and what sort of person this woman is who is touching Him, that she is a sinner" (Luke 7:37-39, explanation added).

Then we see in verses 47-48, Jesus rebuked the Pharisee: **"For this reason I say to you, her sins, which are many, have been forgiven, for she loved much; but he who is forgiven little, loves little." Then He said to her, "Your sins have been forgiven."**

We have taught on the doctrine of worship in the first session, now let us close out the class with an example of worship, and draw some conclusions for our own lives.

The woman in the above story was worshiping Jesus. There is no doubt about her love and devotion to Him, for she worshiped Him with that which was of much value to her; her alabaster vial of perfume, and she not only poured out that perfume on Jesus, but her heart as well.

There is a lesson to learn from this story that can apply directly to those of us who have been overeating. The lesson is this: the woman in this story used in the worship of God that which she had previously used in the acts of sin. She took that alabaster jar of perfume, that which she had used in the deception of her past life, and to gratify her own flesh, and poured it out at Jesus' feet and worshiped Him with it.

Let us learn and apply this lesson in our own lives. It is possible for us to use food, that which we have formerly used to gratify our flesh, in the worship of God. There are many ways to do this, but the key to it all is simply experiencing the love, grace and forgiveness of Jesus Christ. Sinners who are forgiven must love much. And as we experience His grace and compassion our hearts long to worship Him. We want to use that which we formerly used in sin, in the worship of Him who has forgiven us much.

When was the last time you poured out your heart to Jesus, in loving worship of Him who died on the cross to pay for your sins? When is the last time you wept tears of love and repentance to Him who poured out His life for you? Well next time you visit the cross, take some food with you, maybe a meal that you will give up for Him, maybe a sack of groceries given to some poor people, and pour out to Him that which was formerly used for sin and for self.

Hand out question sheets for next week's lesson. Close in prayer.

Handout Questions for Group Discussion
Week 5

Day 16
Question 1. How does the enemy try to tempt us?

Question 2. Why is it vital to have the word of God living in us?

Question 3. According to 1 Corinthians 10:13, should we expect temptation? Is any temptation unique to you?

Day 17
Question 4. What is genuine brokenness?

Question 5. Why must we see the sinfulness of our sin?

Day 18
Question 6. What "keeps" us in bondage to the sin of overeating?

Question 7. How does the truth set us free?

Day 19
Question 8. Where does God take us in order to see that only He can free us?

Question 9. What is the root of our sin?

Question 10. What does it mean to cry out to God?

Day 20
Question 11. According to Leviticus 26:13, what has God already accomplished for us? What is the result? (walk w/God, walk free, walk w/dignity)

Week Five

7:00-7:05:
Call to Order and Opening Prayer

7:05-7:25:
Teaching: Overcoming Temptation (1 Peter 5:8-11).

7:25-7:30:
Small break and reorganize into small groups

7:30-7:55:
Small Group Interaction

7:55-8:05:
Coming back together, singing two to three songs

8:05-8:15:
Teaching and Challenge: Overcoming Temptation and Sin - Illustrated
(Psalm 18:37-40).

Overcoming Temptation

Be of sober spirit, be on the alert. Your adversary, the devil, prowls around like a roaring lion, seeking someone to devour. But resist him, firm in your faith, knowing that the same experiences of suffering are being accomplished by your brethren who are in the world. After you have suffered for a little while, the God of all grace, who called you to His eternal glory in Christ, will Himself perfect, confirm, strengthen and establish you. To Him be dominion forever and ever. Amen" (1 Peter 5:8-11).

Helps for teachers:
This passage shows us that we not only have a traitor within (our own deceitful heart and stubborn flesh) but we have a deceiver without (the devil).

The devil is called our "adversary" as he is our opponent and our enemy. He is described as a "roaring lion" because of his fierce strength. A human being is not able to withstand the strength of a lion.

The way this lion-devil has sought to devour us in the past is through lies and deception. Just as he did in the Garden of Eden, he holds out food to our minds as that which is pleasing to the eye. He lies to us that food will ultimately satisfy us, will comfort us when we are sad or depressed, will provide us friendship when we are lonely, and will give us excitement when we are bored. But food is not designed to fill emptiness in our hearts and the devil is lying when he deceives us in this manner. For many years I was unable to overcome his lies; they seemed too powerful for me. Indeed, every human being who fights the battle on his own against the devil will lose.

Martin Luther wrote of the power of the lion-devil in his famous song, *A Mighty Fortress is our God*. Part of one verse says,

> "For still our ancient foe doth seek to work us woe;
> His craft and power are great, and, armed with cruel hate,
> On earth is not his equal.
> Words & Music: Martin Luther (1483-1546).

Well, what then are we to do with this very strong tempter who seeks to devour us?

"Resist him, firm in your faith" (1 Peter 5:9).

When the devil lies about the benefits of turning to food for issues of the heart, we are to resist him. We are to resist him when he presents pictures to our minds of how good it would feel to indulge our flesh. And when he tempts us with our favorite food, and we are not hungry, we are to resist him.

The Christian life is much about resisting the devil and his attempts at seducing us away from Christ. It seems that he has an unending arsenal of temptations to throw at us to divert us away from Jesus. The Bible tells us to resist him.

When we resist the cravings of our flesh and the seductions of the devil, there will inevitably be pain and suffering involved. That is why the Bible warns us of the suffering that is inevitably involved in resisting the devil, and encourages us to persist through the suffering and find the strength of God.

"But resist him, firm in your faith, knowing that the same experiences of suffering are being accomplished by your brethren who are in the world. After you have suffered for a little while, the God of all grace, who called you to His eternal glory in Christ, will Himself perfect, confirm, strengthen and establish you" (verses 9-10).

It is important for teachers to help the class understand that there is suffering involved in denying our flesh, in crucifying it daily. The Bible does not deny this suffering, but rather encourages us to persist through it and promises that if we do we will find grace and strength from God. Diet gurus today, unfamiliar with the cross, try to eliminate any suffering involved in losing weight. But we know that this is simply not true. Pain and suffering are part of the Christian life for many reasons.

Help the class see that the experience of receiving grace from God, and being strengthened and established by Him, is worth the suffering that comes from resisting the devil. This experience of receiving life-giving strength and grace from God is what makes us different than the moralists who would teach us to "just say no." We don't just say no, we say resist the devil, suffer for a little while, and then be ready to experience the blessing of receiving God's grace, strength, and comfort which will more than make up for the pain of denying the flesh and resisting the devil.

If we ask the class, "Who among you wants to be perfected, confirmed, strengthened and established by God?" we would most likely get a positive response from one hundred percent of the audience. Well, in order to receive these blessings we must first resist the devil and go through a time of suffering in the flesh. This is normal; it is experienced by every Christian (1 Peter 5:9), but it is temporary and is followed shortly thereafter by the grace, comfort, and strength of Almighty God.

Though no human being is equal to the strength of the devil, there is One who has fought the lion and has overcome. We cannot overcome the devil in our own strength but Jesus can, and did. On the cross he defeated satan for us, and is able even now to give us strength to overcome as well. Martin Luther wrote of this power in Jesus:

Did we in our strength confide, our striving would be losing;
Were not the right Man on our side, the Man of God's own choosing:
Dost ask who that may be? Christ Jesus, it is He;
Lord Sabbaoth, His Name, from age to age the same,
And He must win the battle.

Day 16

Question 1. What is the enemy's purpose in tempting us?

Every temptation for us is designed by the enemy of our souls to
cause us to disobey God, and to bypass our own cross. Satan's
design is for us to give in and disobey rather than to resist and offer
our bodies a living sacrifice; to indulge our flesh, rather than
crucify it.

Question 2. Why is it vital to have the word of God living in us?

It is through the application of biblical principles in our lives that
we overcome the evil one (1 John 2:14). This is a vital point, for
we are unable to overcome the devil in our own strength, yet God's
Word actuating us provides victory. The Word of God "living in us"
is more than just reading the Bible, memorizing Scripture, doing
Bible studies; in order for the Word to live in us we must act upon
what we read. As we apply the truths we learn, they take up resi-
dence in our hearts. Psalm 111:10 is a perfect verse to teach here,
for it tells us that it is through the "doing" of God's Word that we
gain understanding, not just the reading, studying or memorizing
of it.

Question 3. According to 1 Corinthians 10:13, should we expect temptation? Is any temptation unique to you?

The Bible tells us that temptation is part of the Christian's experience, and that all temptation is common to Christians. Though
we can have a certain sin that "easily besets" us (Hebrews 12:1),
yet temptation to all sin is common to all people everywhere. One
of the tools of the devil is to make us feel isolated, and to get the

distorted sense that "I am the only one who struggles so hard with this." No, temptation is a common and normal experience among those who are the enemies of the devil.

Day 17

Question 4. What is genuine brokenness?

Genuine brokenness is that experience of life whereby we come to the complete end of ourselves, and where we become desperate for God. A broken person has lost his sinful pride, his self-absorption, his self-confidence. He or she has sensed the reality of the total futility of life apart from Christ, and they begin longing and craving for God as the deer pants for the water. The broken person experiences the nearness of God, and the power of His grace to heal and restore. **"The LORD is near to the brokenhearted and saves those who are crushed in spirit" (Psalm 34:18).**

Question 5. Why must we see the sinfulness of our sin?

It is important that we see the sinfulness of our sin so that we might truly turn away from it and begin to develop a hatred for it. Sin that appears ugly and disgusting can be turned away from; whereas sin that is still viewed as beneficial will have a strong drawing influence on us.

Day 18

Question 6. What "keeps" us in bondage to the sin of overeating?

Sin and deception go hand in hand, so that we never sin unless we are first deceived. Believing lies keeps us in bondage, whereas forsaking them and believing the truth sets us free.

Question 7. How does the truth set us free?

The truth sets us free by enabling us to forsake the lies and deception that enslave the soul.

Day 19

Question 8. What is the root of our sin?

> The root of our sin is the heart. Jesus said, **"But the things that proceed out of the mouth come from the heart, and those defile the man. For out of the heart come evil thoughts, murders, adulteries, fornications, thefts, false witness, slanders. These are the things which defile the man; but to eat with unwashed hands does not defile the man"** (Matthew 15:18-20).

This is important to understand because so many in the diet craze industry either don't recognize overeating as sin, or they can't identify the origin of bad habits. The answer from Scripture is that sin comes from my heart. The world mixes things up and basically teaches that sin is external whereas salvation is internal. They would say that sin is that which happens TO me; my bad upbringing, my early abuses, the bad way my environment has treated me, etc. whereas redemption is within; that is, I just need to experience my own self-actualization, work on my self-esteem, build my self up, etc...

All of this is contrary to truth. In reality, sin is internal and salvation is external. Sin comes from my heart, is part of my spiritual DNA and I have no body to blame for it but myself. Whereas salvation is external, it comes to me through Jesus Christ and His Word.

Question 9. What does it mean to cry out to God?

> The first step to calling out to the Lord the proper way is to humble ourselves. It is to cry to the Lord as a sinner, one who is ashamed of his or her life. The one who calls to the Lord in humility is heard by God. James 4:7 says, **"God opposes the proud, but gives grace to the humble."**

> The second step to calling out to the Lord in the proper way is to repent. Some call to the Lord but they continue on in their sin. Repentance is recognizing that my sin is dishonoring to the Lord and that it will never satisfy me. Instead of turning to sin I now turn to the Lord as the One who alone can meet my need. Jeremiah

2:13 says, **"For My people have committed two evils: They have forsaken Me, the fountain of living waters, and hewn themselves cisterns–broken cisterns that can hold no water."** In repentance, we turn away from the "broken cisterns" and turn back to the Lord who is the Fountain of Living Waters.

The third step to calling out to the Lord in the proper way is to submit to biblical authority and seek help from other believers. Going to church is indispensable, for there I have my soul fed from God's Word, I am challenged and encouraged by other believers, and I find grace. Some people think they can be independent of the body of believers called church, but in so doing they are attempting to separate the Head from the body. God works in His church, Christ is the Head of the body, and His presence is there among His members. **"Obey those who rule over you, and be submissive, for they watch out for your souls, as those who must give account. Let them do so with joy and not with grief, for that would be unprofitable for you"** (Hebrews 13:17). **"And let us consider one another in order to stir up love and good works, not forsaking the assembling of ourselves together, as is the manner of some, but exhorting one another, and so much the more as you see the Day approaching"** (Hebrews 10:24-25).

Day 20

Question 10. According to Leviticus 26:13, what has God already accomplished for us? What is the result?

God both breaks the power of sin in our lives and removes the shame and the guilt of sin. The verse says that He "breaks the bars of our yoke" which is descriptive way of stating that He breaks the power of sin in our lives. The picture is of two oxen, yoked together in servitude, and going the same direction. It reminds us of our time in sin, when we were literally yoked together with sin and served the lusts of our flesh. But God has broken this power in our lives.

And not only has He broken the power of sin He has also remove the guilt and shame of sin. The verse says that He "enables us to walk with our heads held high" which again is a descriptive picture of a man without guilt or shame.

At the cross, Jesus took our sin upon Himself and died to pay the penalty of it. In so doing, He removed the sin burden and the yoke of the law, enabling us to be rid of shame and guilt for our past sin. It is extremely valuable to see that the power of sin, as well as the guilt and shame of sin, has been broken.

8:05-8:15 pm:
Final Teaching and Challenge: Overcoming Sin

"I pursued my enemies and overtook them, and I did not turn back until they were consumed. I shattered them, so that they were not able to rise; they fell under my feet. For You have girded me with strength for battle; You have subdued under me those who rose up against me. You have also made my enemies turn their backs to me, and I destroyed those who hated me" (Psalm 18:37-40).

This passage in Psalms presents to us a picture of what it takes to truly overcome temptation and sin. It shows us David as he goes on the offensive to destroy his enemies completely, and it almost appears as if it is "overkill" for he not only "pursued and overtook" them, not only "consumed" them but he also "shattered" them so that they could not rise again.

Becoming successful in the battle with weight loss should not be simply stopping our overeating, we should go on to take the offensive in the battle and look at ways we can ensure the defeat of our flesh and how we might "crush and shatter" the power of temptation in our lives. We are to be proactive in this battle, developing strategies that ensure our victory, and making sure every avenue of temptation is dealt with ahead of time so that we won't fall under "surprise attack."

The Kingdom of God is an offensive (not defensive) kingdom, and we are to pursue our enemies just as David did, and we are to crush and shatter them so that we are assured of victory over them. Matthew 16:18 confirms that the Kingdom of God is offensive in nature, showing Christians breaking through the defensive gates of the evil one and rescuing the captives.

Challenge the class to look for ways they can develop an effective battle strategy against our enemies of overeating and laziness, and all other sins, helping them to seek God for grace to implement their strategies. Challenge them to get creative and to allow their imaginations to run wild with ways to win the battle.

Finally, it would be important to close with the truth contained in verse 40 of Psalm 18, for if we are victorious in anything it is only because God fights for us. David noted that God made his enemies turn their backs and run from him, so that in reality the battle was the Lord's and victory belonged to Him alone. We can and should develop our plans for defeating sin, but ultimately the outcome belongs to God. This makes us dependent upon Him.

Hand out question sheets for next week's lesson. Close in prayer.

Handout Questions for Group Discussion
Week 6

Day 21
Question 1. According to Numbers 21:4-10 and Hebrews 12:1-3, what is the cure for sin?

Question 2. What does it mean to fix our eyes on Christ in Hebrews 12:2, and consider Him in verse 3? What is the result of considering Jesus?

Day 22
Question 3. What should be our motivation to offer our bodies as a living sacrifice? How are we radically transformed? (Romans 12:1-2).

Question 4. What is the source for renewing/cleansing our minds? (Ephesians 5:26).

Day 23
Question 5. Compare John 7:37-39 and Ephesians 6:18. What is the correlation between drinking from Christ and being filled with the Holy Spirit?

Question 6. What does it mean to be an exclusive drinker? (Psalm 87:7).

Day 24
Question 7. From Matthew 26:40-41, what is Jesus' warning to us & how does that apply to our eating?

Question 8. Read I Corinthians 10:12. What is the relationship between trusting in ourselves and falling into sin?

Day 25
Question 9. What is the real purpose of **The Lord's Table**? (Isaiah 40).

Week Six

7:00-7:05:
Call to Order and Opening Prayer

7:05-7:25:
Teaching: Grace! (Titus 2:11-14).

7:25-7:30:
Small break and reorganize into small groups

7:30-7:55:
Small Group Interaction

7:55-8:05:
Coming back together, singing two to three songs

8:05-8:15:
Teaching and Challenge: Grace Illustrated (Ezra 9:5-9).

Grace

[11] For the grace of God has appeared, bringing salvation to all men, [12] instructing us to deny ungodliness and worldly desires and to live sensibly, righteously and godly in the present age, [13] looking for the blessed hope and the appearing of the glory of our great God and Savior, Christ Jesus, [14] who gave Himself for us to redeem us from every lawless deed, and to purify for Himself a people for His own possession, zealous for good deeds" (Titus 2:11-14).

Helps for teachers:
The grace of God not only saves us from sin's guilt and condemnation, but it also sanctifies us (sets us apart) from sin's power. This is the beauty of God's grace; it saves, and it sanctifies.

This sanctifying influence of God's grace is taught in verse 12 above: "instructing us to deny ungodliness and worldly desires." It is critical to understand that it is God's grace, and God's grace alone, that is able to set us apart from sin, that teaches us to deny ungodliness, and instructs us in sensible and self-controlled living. God's grace is what enables us to lose weight and keep it off, doing it with the right attitude and for the right purpose (to glorify God).

The diet gurus today have a list of things we must do, and many of their systems are very much like a religion with many rules and regulations. Yet these systems that are man-made and are man-centered have no power to restrain the lusts of the flesh. Only the grace of God is stronger than the pull of sin.

It is important that the class understands that the grace of God does the following things:
The grace of God:

- Brings life to those who are dead in sins and trespasses (Ephesians 2:8-9).
- Grants repentance to those who are in the devil's trap (2 Timothy 2:25-26).
- Changes the hearts of men and women (Ezekiel 36:26).
- Crucifies the "old man" (the sinful nature) and makes us "new creations" in Christ (Galatians 2:20).
- Frees up the "will" and enables us to "do" God's will (Philippians 2:13).
- Teaches us to deny ungodliness, and to live sensibly and in self-control (Titus 2:11-13).

Titus 2:14 tells us that God's intention in sending Jesus to die for us was that He would "redeem us" and "purify us." Again, these are terms that describe "salvation" (redemption from sin) and "sanctification" (purification from sins). Both of these aspects are accomplished only by God's grace.

In opposition to God's grace are our own works, rules placed upon us by false religious systems and popular diets, vows and promises to "do better" and our own "will power." Those who have struggled long, have made vows and decisions only to break them, and are now at the point of having no hope of ever being free, are prime candidates for the grace of God. Once someone comes to the end of themselves, they are ready to receive the amazing grace of God which will enable and empower them to deny their flesh and to walk uprightly.

Grace is truly amazing, not only in forgiving our sins and removing our guilt and shame, but also in teaching and empowering us to deny unrighteousness (overeating) and to live with discipline and victory in our lives.

Help the class to see that it is not new vows that are needed, that it is not a new diet they need to try, but rather they need God's grace.

Day 21

Question 1. According to Numbers 21:4-10 and Hebrews 12:1-3, what is the cure for sin?

> According to Numbers 21:4-10 and Hebrews 12:1-3, the cure for sin is to focus on Jesus Christ. The whole point of the story in Numbers 21: 4-10 is to show that the cure for sin is in the gospel of Jesus Christ. It would be good for the teacher to bring in John 3:14-15 here, which is Jesus' explanation of the Numbers 21 passage, to show the connection between the cure for the snake-bitten Israelites and our cure for sin.

Question 2. What does it mean to fix our eyes on Christ in Hebrews 12:2, and consider Him in verse 3? What is the result of considering Jesus?

> This is a question for discussion. Encourage the students to interact here and to discuss these questions, coming to conclusions that would benefit the whole class.

Day 22

Question 3. What should be our motivation to offer our bodies as a living sacrifice? How are we radically transformed? (Romans 12:1-2).

> The proper motivation to offering God our bodies is in light of the grace He has shown us in Christ. As God gives us grace, which turns our hearts away from sin and to His Son, we begin to love Him as He first loved us. Out of the grace He shows us, we desire to present our bodies to Him as a living sacrifice.

We are radically transformed (Greek, "metamorphoo") by renewing our minds. It is for this reason that Christians should be warned about fad diet programs and diet gurus who propagate information in huge amounts, who sound like experts, who claim special knowledge, but who, in reality, are actually contributing to the problem of gluttony and laziness by disseminating information that is untrue. Christians need to understand that the condition of being overweight is from the sin problem of overeating, and that the solution is through repenting faith in Christ. The problem is not that we combine our foods wrongly, or that we eat the wrong kinds of foods (for all foods have been declared clean by Jesus). It is sometimes very difficult to overcome the very loud and deceptive voice that is coming from the diet craze industry, which is why at **The Lord's Table** we hold closely to Scripture, which is the truth that sets us free.

Question 4. What is the source for renewing/cleansing our minds? (Ephesians 5:26).

> The source for renewing our minds is God's Word, and the source for cleansing our hearts and minds is God's Word.

Day 23

Question 5. Compare John 7:37-39 and Ephesians 5:18-19. What is the correlation between drinking from Christ and being filled with the Holy Spirit?

> The correlation between drinking from Christ and being filled with the Spirit is that as we receive the Living Water from Jesus, the Holy Spirit flows out of our hearts. Ephesians 5:18 describes one who drinks in the Spirit of God, and verse 19 describes the Spirit of God flowing out of us as we speak to each other in songs, hymns and spiritual songs.
>
> The main point in both of these passages is that the Living Water satisfies us and the wine of the Holy Spirit controls us. A person who is satisfied in Christ and controlled by the Holy Spirit is a

person free from bondage to sin. Overeating is overcome, not by a diet, pill, or gimmick, but through satisfying our hearts in Jesus and experiencing the control of the Holy Spirit.

Question 6. What does it mean to be an exclusive drinker? (Psalm 87:7).

Being an exclusive drinker means that my only source of satisfaction and life comes through Jesus Christ. We are not saying that we can't receive joy and delight in our spouses, or in our work, or that we can't have hobbies, etc. What we are really referring to from Psalm 87:7 is a man or woman free from habitual sin. We are no longer "drinking" from other sources for we have discovered life-giving water in Jesus.

Day 24

Question 7. What is Jesus' warning to us in Matthew 26:40-41, and how does that apply to our eating?

In Matthew 26:40-41, Jesus instructs us to the fact that we have weak flesh and warns us to be vigilant against giving in to sin. Verse 41 is an excellent description of the believer, for our spirits are willing to resist and avoid all sin, but the flesh is weak and can fall easily.

Especially is this warning important when it comes to our eating habits. With other sins such as drunkenness, pornography, drug addiction, etc. the source can be "radically amputated" (Matthew 5:29-30) so that we cannot physically get our hands on that which tempts us. But when it comes to overeating issues we cannot forsake food entirely, so the warning to be on guard against temptation is extremely practical.

We must understand that temptation to overeat (and many other sins) will be with us for life. Therefore, we must be vigilant to watch for them, and when we sense them coming upon us, to run to prayer immediately. We recognize that God is able to **"deliver the needy when he cries for help, the afflicted also, and him who has no helper"(Psalm 72:12),** and so we "watch" for temptation and we "pray" when we see it coming.

Question 8. What is the relationship between trusting in ourselves and falling into sin? (1 Corinthians 10:12)

> The person who trusts in himself hasn't yet learned the deceitfulness of his own heart, the weakness of his flesh, nor the power and craftiness of the devil. Because they are ignorant of these very powerful enemies, they can be deceived easily and are just one slip away from a fall into sin.

> The person who has experienced the weakness of their resolves not to sin, and the powerful onslaughts of temptation from the devil, knows that he cannot rely on himself to withstand the force of temptation and sin. Instead, he knows to run to God immediately, beseeching Him for help, clinging to Him for grace.

We want the students to really understand this issue. This is also the value of a testimony, where someone can share that they tried to be free from sin on their own, or through diets or pills, etc. but could never find freedom from the power of temptation. But through Christ, and the grace received in Him we can be free.

Day 25

Question 9. What is the real purpose of **The Lord's Table**? (Isaiah 40).

> The real purpose of this course is to assist us in seeing God accurately, and to loving Him supremely. If the Holy Spirit opens our eyes to see the vastness, majesty and glory of God, as well as His love and power and grace, then the natural response in the heart of the believer is worship and love of God. In other words, this course in not just about ceasing sinful behavior; it is about helping us to love God.

8:05-8:15 pm:
Final Teaching and Challenge: Grace Illustrated

"But at the evening offering I arose from my humiliation, even with my garment and my robe torn, and I fell on my knees and stretched out my hands to the LORD my God; and I said, "O my God, I am

ashamed and embarrassed to lift up my face to You, my God, for our iniquities have risen above our heads and our guilt has grown even to the heavens. Since the days of our fathers to this day we have been in great guilt, and on account of our iniquities we, our kings and our priests have been given into the hand of the kings of the lands, to the sword, to captivity and to plunder and to open shame, as it is this day. But now for a brief moment grace has been shown from the LORD our God, to leave us an escaped remnant and to give us a peg in His holy place, that our God may enlighten our eyes and grant us a little reviving in our bondage. For we are slaves; yet in our bondage our God has not forsaken us, but has extended lovingkindness to us in the sight of the kings of Persia, to give us reviving to raise up the house of our God, to restore its ruins and to give us a wall in Judah and Jerusalem" (Ezra 9:5-9).

Ezra chapter 9 is an amazing chapter that shows the power and effectiveness of grace. The Israelites had been sinning by their intermarrying of pagan wives and in their whoredom of pursuing relationships with other nations. As a result of their sins they were taken captive to Babylon and subjected to forced labor and harsh conditions.

But the predicted time of their captivity came to a close and as they returned to Jerusalem they were reminded of their sin that sent them into captivity, and Ezra initiates a national repentance and reformation.

In the passage above, Ezra is praying to God on behalf of the people, listing their sins and confessing them. But amidst the recollection of the sins of the people and the captivity that came about as a result, He recalls the grace of God and the effects of that grace. He says in verses 8 and 9.

"But now for a brief moment grace has been shown from the LORD our God, to leave us an escaped remnant and to give us a peg in His holy place, that our God may enlighten our eyes and grant us a little reviving in our bondage. For we are slaves; yet in our bondage our God has not forsaken us, but has extended lovingkindness to us in the sight of the kings of Persia, to give us reviving to raise up the house of our God, to restore its ruins and to give us a wall in Judah and Jerusalem."

In these two verses we are shown the diamond of Gods grace, set to the black backdrop of sin. Sin always brings bondage, captivity and death (see John 8:34), but grace is that which revives, enlightens, and frees us from bondage.

We want to show the class the amazing power of God's grace. It was by God's grace that the Israelites were set free from captivity to Babylon, and it is by God's grace that we are set free from captivity to sin. It was by God's grace that He revived Israel when they were languishing in Babylon, and it by God's grace that we are revived from long periods of sin and rebellion. It was by God's grace that He enabled the returned captives to restore and rebuild the ruins of Jerusalem and the temple, and it is by God's grace that we begin to rebuild and restore lives ruined by sin. Grace, grace, grace, it's amazing to those who have experienced it, and who experience it on a daily basis.

Close with the challenge to seek God for grace, and to know that when we are released from captivity and begin to rebuild and restore lives that we have received His grace in abundance. **"But the Law entered so that the offense might abound. But where sin abounded, grace did much more abound, so that as sin has reigned to death, even so grace might reign through righteousness to eternal life by Jesus Christ our Lord" (Romans 5:20-21).**

God's grace saved me from all wrong
God's grace gave my heart a new song

God's grace turned my heart from sin
God's grace changed me from within

God's grace removed my guilt and shame
God's grace enables me to glorify His Name

Now I come to you, with God's grace in my heart
And ask of you from sin, by God's grace, to depart

(A testimony of Grace, by Mike Cleveland)

Hand out question sheets for next week's lesson. Close in prayer.

Handout Questions for Group Discussion
Week 7

Day 26
Question 1. What are the links in the accident chain mentioned in James 1:13-15?

Question 2. How can we break the chain at the first link?

Day 27
Question 3. What is the flesh? What is the Spirit? (Galatians 5:17).

Question 4. How do we walk in the Spirit? (Galatians 5:16-26).

Question 5. From Romans 8:5-9 List the differences between the mind set on the spirit and the mind set on the flesh.

Day 28
Question 6. From 1 John 1:5-7, what is the result of walking in the light?

Question 7. What does it mean to be a new creation in Christ? (2 Corinthians 5:17). Are you living as a new creation?

Day 29
Question 8. Read 2 Peter 3:17-18. What is vital to our spiritual growth?

Day 30
Question 9. What two factors must be present in order to obtain great gain? (1 Timothy 6:6).

Question 10. Read Philippians 4:11-12. Is our contentment dependent on our circumstances?

Week Seven

7:00-7:05:
Call to Order and Opening Prayer

7:05-7:25:
Teaching: Humility and Grace (James 4:6-10).

7:25-7:30:
Small break and reorganize into small groups

7:30-7:55:
Small Group Interaction

7:55-8:05:
Coming back together, singing two to three songs

8:05-8:15:
Teaching and Challenge: Illustration of Grace

Humility and Grace

⁶"But He gives a greater grace. Therefore it says, 'GOD IS OPPOSED TO THE PROUD, BUT GIVES GRACE TO THE HUMBLE.' ⁷Submit therefore to God. Resist the devil and he will flee from you. ⁸Draw near to God and He will draw near to you. Cleanse your hands, you sinners; and purify your hearts, you double-minded. ⁹Be miserable and mourn and weep; let your laughter be turned into mourning and your joy to gloom. ¹⁰Humble yourselves in the presence of the Lord, and He will exalt you"(James 4:6-10).

Last week we studied the power of God's grace to free us from habitual sin. This week we want to see how to get that grace from God which will enable us to break free from overeating. The way we get grace from God, according to James 4:6-10 is to humble ourselves, for **"God gives grace to the humble."**

Habitual sin not only hardens our hearts but it also makes us prideful, arrogant, and puffed up. In turn, pride goes before a fall, so there is a never ending cycle of pride, sin, pride, sin. This pride causes God to "oppose" (verse 6) or resist us. The word "opposed" in verse 6 means to arrange oneself against, in a military fashion, so as to mightily oppose. In short, it is a hard thing to have the living God in opposition to us, and victory will not come into the life of one whom God opposes.

This cycle of sin/pride/sin/pride, which results in the opposition of Almighty God, requires grace in the heart in order to break free. And grace comes into the heart when we humble ourselves in the presence of the Lord.

The word "humble" in verse 10 is defined by the NASB exhaustive concordance as "to depress; figuratively to humiliate (in condition or heart): - abase, bring low, humble (self)."

It is this lowering of ourselves in the presence of God that brings grace into our hearts. As we bring ourselves low, acknowledging our sins, admitting our failures, confessing our guilt, repenting of an exalted view of self, the kindness and grace of God comes into our hearts. And grace picks us up, strengthens our hearts, and enables our victory.

Challenge the class to take some time of quietness to humble themselves before the Lord, to confess any and every sin, to acknowledge any exalted view of self, and to seek God for grace.
After this moment of silent self-humbling in the presence of God, close this session by reading these selected verses:

"When pride comes, then comes dishonor, but with the humble is wisdom" (Proverbs 11:2).

"A man's pride will bring him low, but a humble spirit will obtain honor" (Proverbs 29:23).

"But if you will not listen to it, My soul will sob in secret for such pride; and my eyes will bitterly weep and flow down with tears, because the flock of the LORD has been taken captive" (Jeremiah 13:17).

"Moreover, the pride of Israel testifies against him, and Israel and Ephraim stumble in their iniquity; Judah also has stumbled with them" (Hosea 5:5).

"In the wilderness He fed you manna which your fathers did not know, that He might humble you and that He might test you, to do good for you in the end" (Deuteronomy 8:16).

"He leads the humble in justice, and He teaches the humble His way" (Psalm 25:9).

Day 26

Question 1. What are the links in the accident chain mentioned in James 1:13-15?

> The links in the accident chain from James 1:13-15 include:
> Temptation
> Being "carried away" and enticed
> Lust
> Sin
> Death

Question 2. How can we break the chain at the first link?

> This is a question for open discussion and many different students should present their views so that the group can benefit from the different members.

Day 27

Question 3. What is the flesh? What is the Spirit? (Galatians 5:17).

> The flesh is that part of us that is unredeemed (Romans 8:23). It is the "residue" of the "old man" that was put to death in conversion. All believers have flesh, or "that which remains of wickedness" (James 1:21).
>
> The Spirit, in this context, is the Holy Spirit of God.

Question 4. How do we walk in the Spirit? (Galatians. 5:16-26).

Walking in the Spirit is better caught than taught. It has to do with fellowshiping with the Spirit of God, of communion, of friendship, of intimacy and delight. The effects of this walking in the Spirit are that we do not gratify the lusts of our flesh. Enoch walked with God "and was no more" for God took Him. In a spiritual sense the same is true of us; when we walk with God, we are no more, that is when we walk with God we do not gratify the lusts of our flesh.

It is for this reason that we at **The Lord's Table** do not teach people to simply stop overeating. Rather, we want to teach the importance of fellowshiping with God, of walking in the Spirit, of developing a strong and vibrant relationship with Christ, and the byproduct will be the ceasing of sinful patterns of thought and behavior.

These things need to be taught over and over again as it is very easy for Christians to lose the fellowship and intimacy of the Spirit of God by becoming focused on other things, or to quench the fire of the Holy Spirit by continual giving in to the flesh.

Question 5. From Romans 8:5-9 list the differences between the mind set on the Spirit and the mind set on the flesh.

- The mind set on the flesh is death, but the mind set on the Spirit is life and peace.
- The mind set on the flesh is hostile to God and cannot subject itself to the law of God, but the mind set on the Spirit is in subjection to God.
- The mind set on the flesh cannot please God but the mind set on the Spirit is pleasing to God.

(Some of the above answers are "positive inference" from the negative. That is, if the negative is true, the opposite positive is also true, though it may not be clearly stated in the text.)

Day 28

Question 6. From 1 John 1:5-7, what is the result of walking in the light?

> There are two results of walking in the light which are stated in 1 John 1:5-7. They are:
> > Fellowship with other Christians.
> > Cleansing from all sin.
>
> This makes sense as Christians are those who walk in the light, and if we walk in the light we will have fellowship together. The light is that which purges the darkness and cleanses dirty spots, and as we walk in the light we are cleansed from sin.
>
> Again there is an importance in this passage of Scripture that calls us to walking in the Spirit, or walking in the light, rather than just stopping overeating. If we will purposefully learn to fellowship with Christ, through the Holy Spirit, we will find sweet fellowship with others who are doing the same, and we will be cleansed from habitual sin.

Question 7. What does it mean to be a new creation in Christ? (2 Corinthians 5:17). Are you living as a new creation?

> This question is designed for group interaction. The ideas we want to convey are that as new creations in Christ we need to live as such.

Day 29

Question 8. According to 2 Peter 3:17-18, what keeps us from falling away from steadfastness? In other words, how do we persevere?

> Being carried away with error causes us to fall away from steadfastness. So instead, we must grow in grace and knowledge of our Lord and Savior, Jesus Christ. Steadfastness comes from a knowledgeable relationship with Christ that is based upon the implementation of truth in the life.

Day 30

Question 9. According to 1 Timothy 6:6, what two factors must be present in order to obtain great gain?

> Godliness and contentment

Question 10. According to Philippians 4:11-12, should our contentment be dependent on our circumstances?

> Our contentment should not be dependant upon our circumstances; we are called to be content in Christ no matter what. Paul had learned to be content both when hungry and when filled, when he was in need or when he abounded. His heart was happy in Christ no matter what his circumstances. Help the students learn that contentment in Christ should be present even when they are physically hungry. This contentment when hungry truly can be a reality in the life of one who is enjoying a vibrant and growing relationship with Jesus.

8:05-8:15 pm:
Final Teaching and Challenge: Grace Illustrated

"Have this attitude in yourselves which was also in Christ Jesus, who, although He existed in the form of God, did not regard equality with God a thing to be grasped, but emptied Himself, taking the form of a bond-servant, and being made in the likeness of men. Being found in appearance as a man, He humbled Himself by becoming obedient to the point of death, even death on a cross. For this reason also, God highly exalted Him, and bestowed on Him the name which is above every name, so that at the name of Jesus EVERY KNEE WILL BOW, of those who are in heaven and on earth and under the earth" **(Philippians 2:5-10).**

This passage of Scripture presents, as no other passage, what humility truly is. Jesus Christ was and is fully God, equal with the Father, yet He did not cling to His equality but rather lowered Himself to become a man, then lowered Himself further to become a slave, then emptied Himself on the cross to become our Savior and Redeemer. He came from God to Man, from Heaven to earth, from glory to humiliation. He came from the highest of highs and descended to the lowest of lows. And this same attitude is to be in us.

If we are willing to lower ourselves, taking our proper position before God, He will exalt us and lift us up in His time, even as Jesus was highly exalted after the suffering of the cross and given the name which is ABOVE every name, and He will receive the worship of all mankind. God will give us grace in response to our self-humbling, and His grace enables us to walk in victory over the flesh and to live lives of self-control and moderation.

As we focus on the beautiful changes made in lives that are given grace by God, let us remember that purposeful humbling of ourselves is the way to grace, and grace is the way to victory over sin. Grace makes all things beautiful, and self-humbling paves the way for the reception of grace.

Hand out question sheets for next lesson. Close in prayer.

Handout Questions for Group Discussion
Week 8

Day 31

Question 1. List the "3 D's" that are foundational to The Lord's Table course.

Question 2. According to John 6:50-58, what does Jesus promise to those who eat His flesh and drink His blood?

Question 3. According to Ecclesiastes 4:9-12, what are the benefits of accountability?

Day 32

Question 4. When we abide in Christ and He in us, what are the results? (John 15:4-11). How much joy will be ours according to verse 11?

Day 33

Question 5. Read Proverbs 31:10-31. Did this woman exercise?

Question 6. Reflecting on this proverb, what is the purpose of exercise today?

Day 34

Question 7. What is the food by which our hearts are established? (Hebrews 13:9-10).

Day 35

Question 8. Define perseverance from
       Romans 5:1-5,
       2 Timothy 3:10-17
       Galatians 6:9

Question 9. What is the definition of progress in TLT? (paragraph 7)

Question 10. Read Romans 5:3-5. What are the stages we must go through in order to have hope?

Week Eight

7:00-7:05:
Call to Order and Opening Prayer

7:05-7:25:
Teaching: Perseverance (Selected Scripture - see below).

7:25-7:30:
Short break and reorganize into small groups

7:30-7:55:
Small Group Interaction

7:55-8:05:
Coming back together, singing two to three songs

8:05-8:15:
Teaching and Challenge: Illustration of Perseverance

Perseverance

This is the end of the seventh week and we are over half-way through the study. About this time some people are really losing weight, some are struggling, but all are in need of perseverance. At this time in the course it may help to paraphrase the material on Day 22 in **The Lord's Table** manual and follow that with a Scriptural study on perseverance.

"I love this metamorphosis, and don't ever want to go back to crawling in the mud. How about you? This is Day 22 for you, and most people begin to see real changes happening by now. But also about this time the devil begins stomping his feet and throwing a temper tantrum over his captives leaving. Some people begin having dreams of food they've never had before, others find that suddenly temptation is all around them, and still others find that food becomes available where it never was before, others become critical and irritable because their flesh is craving and they are denying it. Hang in there. The hardest part for most people is the first few months until good and godly habits replace the previous bad ones. I'm telling you this as a warning that things may get harder before they get easier, and to be forewarned is to be forearmed."

Have the class look up and read with you the following passages of Scripture, making a few comments about them, time permitting:

> Luke 8:11-15
> Romans 2:5-7
> Romans 5:3-5
> Romans 15:4-6
> Ephesians 6:18
> 2 Thessalonians 1:4
> 1 Timothy 6:11
> 2 Peter 1:5-8

The challenge should be to persevere, not only through the course but also through our entire lives. There are forces that would seek to prevent our perseverance; we must seek the Lord to lead us not into temptation (Matthew 6:13), to keep us from falling (Jude 1:24) and to keep us safe and bring us home at last. We can be thankful that Jesus promised to lose none of His own (John 6:39) and one of the ways that He keeps us in Him is to instruct us in the need to persevere.

Day 31

Question 1. List the "3 D's" that are foundational to The Lord's Table course.

> Delight Your Soul
> Discipline Your Body
> Develop Accountability

Question 2. According to John 6:50-58, what does Jesus promise to those who eat His flesh and drink His blood?

> Jesus promises LIFE to those who eat His flesh and drink His blood.

Question 3. According to Ecclesiastes 4:9-12, what are the benefits of accountability?

> Spiritual fruit (verse 9)
> Spiritual restoration (verse 10)

Spiritual zeal (verse 11)
Spiritual protection (verse 12)

Day 32

Question 4. When we abide in Christ and He in us, what are the results? (John 15:4-11). How much joy will be ours according to verse 11?

Day 33

Question 5. Read Proverbs 31:10-31. Did this woman exercise?

Question 6. Reflecting on this proverb, what is one purpose of exercise today?

> This proverb teaches us that exercise is not only to make the body healthy, but also for the purpose of ministry. The woman in Proverbs 31 ministered to and blessed her family by the activities she pursued. It is at this point that the class can learn the value of exercise in that it will inevitably increase ministry capacity. This should be a strong motivator to daily exercise.

Day 34

Question 7. What is the food by which our hearts are established? (Hebrews 13:9-10).

> According to Hebrews 13:9-10, it is the food of grace that establishes our hearts. This is important to understand, for a strong heart enables a disciplined body. When we feed on grace, that is, when we are nourished by it, we become strong soldiers in the battle against our lusts.

Day 35

Question 8. Define perseverance from Romans 5:1-5, 2 Timothy 3:10-17, Galatians 6:9

> Each of these passages describes perseverance in different terms. This is a general discussion question, the purpose of which is to

have the students come to a biblical understanding of, and commit to the importance of, perseverance.

Question 9. What is the definition of progress in **The Lord's Table** Manual? (paragraph 7)

"Progress" should be defined as purposely enjoying the Lord, eating in a disciplined manner every day, making sure we get a moderate amount of exercise, and remaining accountable for these life habits. Remember, as Christians we want to live out the "3 D's: Delight our soul, Discipline our body, Develop Accountability.

There is a reason for this definition of progress. If our goal is only to lose weight, what do we do once we have lost the weight? If we have not developed a change in the way we live our lives, then we will soon be back up in weight, plus some. So our goal is not just to lose weight; but rather it is to live life in a disciplined and self-controlled manner in every area. The by-product of this goal will indeed be weight loss, and the weight loss will be permanent because of the lifestyle change.

So, our definition of "progress" needs to be clarified. Progress for us means that we do not let a day pass without rejoicing our souls in Christ, that each day we eat our food in a planned and self-controlled manner, that we exercise our bodies, and that we are careful to maintain daily accountability with someone. If we purposely live every day in this manner we will lose weight.

Question 10. Read Romans 5:3-5. What are the stages we must go through in order to have hope?

Tribulations
Perseverance
Proven character
Hope

8:05-8:15 pm:
Final Teaching and Challenge: Perseverance Illustrated

When he came, behold, Eli was sitting on his seat by the road eagerly watching, because his heart was trembling for the ark of God. So the man came to tell it in the city, and all the city cried out. When Eli heard the noise of the outcry, he said, "What does the noise of this commotion mean?" Then the man came hurriedly and told Eli. Now Eli was ninety-eight years old, and his eyes were set so that he could not see. The man said to Eli, "I am the one who came from the battle line. Indeed, I escaped from the battle line today." And he said, "How did things go, my son?" Then the one who brought the news replied, "Israel has fled before the Philistines and there has also been a great slaughter among the people, and your two sons also, Hophni and Phinehas, are dead, and the ark of God has been taken." When he mentioned the ark of God, Eli fell off the seat backward beside the gate, and his neck was broken and he died, for he was old and heavy. Thus he judged Israel forty years" (1 Samuel 4:13-18).

Eli serves as a negative illustration of perseverance. He was a priest, called into the service of Yahweh, but somewhere along the line he slipped from his high calling into a life of gratifying his flesh. He and his sons took the fat portions of the offerings for themselves, they gratified themselves with this food, and Eli died as a man who was "old and fat" (1 Samuel 4:18). How opposite this epitaph is from righteous Abraham, who persevered in faith, and died "an old man and full" (or as the NASB has it, "an old man and satisfied with life" Genesis 25:8).

Eli, as he lived his life of pandering to his flesh, began to lose perspective in all areas. God chastised him for not rebuking his sons for their blatant disregard for God's law and their unfaithful ministry. These sons, though priests of Judaism, were "worthless men who did not know the Lord" (1 Samuel 2:12). The failure to confront obvious unrighteousness in his sons shows the weakness of Eli's own character.

When we are seeking to lose weight for the glory of God we must persevere through many trials, through the rebellion of our flesh, through plateaus, and many other obstacles. The glory of God must be our motive, and we must seek the Lord to keep us from falling. There is a strong warning coming from the life of Eli, that those who turn from a life of honoring the Lord will inevitably live a life of indulging the flesh. It is entirely possible that we, too, if we fail to persevere in faith, will die "old and fat."

Hand out questions for next week's lesson. Close in prayer.

Handout Questions for Group Discussion
Week 9

Day 36

1. Psalm 23:1 states "The Lord is my Shepherd". Is this true for you? If it is, then is the second phrase of the verse, "I shall not want," (or lack) true also?

2. According to 2 peter 1:3-4, what has God granted us?

Day 37

3. Romans 6:16-18 teaches that we were once slaves to sin, but are now slaves to righteousness. What does it mean to be a slave to righteousness, specifically as applied to the area of weight loss, eating right, exercise, etc?

4. In 1 Corinthians 6:11, what three things may we expect God's Holy Spirit to do in our lives when we call on the name of the Lord Jesus?

5. According to James 1:22, what is the only correct response to God's Word?

Day 38

6. Read Philippians 3:7-14. What is gained when we pursue Christ? What is the goal of pressing on?

Day 39

7. How does Zephaniah 3:17-19 show us the way to victory?

Day 40

8. How does Luke 17:33 fit in with the idea of our being called to suffer and to die to ourselves?

Week Nine

7:00-7:05:
Call to Order and Opening Prayer

7:05-7:25:
Teaching - Living the Truth (1 John 2:3-6).

7:25-7:30:
Small break and reorganize into small groups

7:30-7:55:
Small Group Interaction

7:55-8:05:
Coming back together, singing two to three songs

8:05-8:15:
Teaching and Challenge - Definition of Living the Truth

Living the Truth

The following article has been taken from one of Mike Cleveland's writings to the online mentors of Setting Captives Free. Mike writes daily Scriptural teachings, challenges and encouragements to the online mentors who volunteer in ministry and this teaching is applicable to mentors and course members alike. Please begin the class today by reading 1 John 2:3-6 and then read the following article:

I wanted to write a note of encouragement and of challenge to you today in hopes that God's Word will be used in your life as it has been in mine lately. I received a note from a student the other day that went something like this:

"No, I am not finding 'freedom' from 'sin' as you would put it. I am a Christian and Christians are different from every other religion in that we have God's forgiveness. You are attempting to make me 'perfect' rather than enforcing the truth that I am forgiven. I am forgiven for all sins, past, present and future. That means that when I sin today, as I know I will, I am forgiven. I have no intention of leaving behind the enjoyment that God gives me freely in eating food, nor the forgiveness that comes by His grace if I overeat."

The man weighs nearly 400 pounds.

Let's examine the Word of God and we will see a big difference between what the above student believed and what Scripture teaches:

"By this we know that we have come to know Him, if we keep His commandments. The one who says, 'I have come to know Him,' and does not keep His commandments, is a liar, and the truth is not in him; but whoever keeps His word, in him the love of God has truly been perfected. By this we know that we are in Him: the one who says he abides in Him ought himself to walk in the same manner as He walked" (1 John 2:3-6).

Friends, God's Word is clear that His kingdom is not about "talk" but about power (1 Corinthians 2:4; 4:19-20)! At Setting Captives Free we are on a mission; a mission to help people to freedom from the self-deception that leaves them in bondage. We are on a mission to help men and women to freedom from sinful bondage, freedom to live without hypocrisy, freedom to truly love Jesus. Our mission is clearly defined; help men and women to acknowledge the truth about themselves and what their lives have been like under deception, help them to turn from all sin, help them to walk in the light of truth.

The passage above in 1 John tells us that there can be a discrepancy between our words and our lives. We can say, "I have come to know Him," that is, profess to be Christians, while our lives evidence that we don't keep His Word. If this is the case then the passage tells us the truth is not in us. In other words, we are living in deception.

This is a very important truth for us to grasp, for there exists a great possibility of self-deception. We are born in this world quite ready to give ourselves the benefit of the doubt. We think we are great, and we wonder why everybody else doesn't agree. This type of thinking shows a deceived heart, for the person who knows what his sinful nature is by birth, who has experienced the deception of his own heart, who has been chewed up by the roaring lion called the Devil, has a proper view of self. He has come out from under the delusion that he is somebody, and he agrees with God that he is sinful by nature and in need of grace to change. This person walks in the light of truth and is not deceived.

Dear mentors, help your students to understand that "our lives speak louder than our words" and to be cautious of saying, "I have come to know Him" if they do not keep his commandments.

Another example is one person who was going through **The Lord's Table** course, losing weight, and providing brilliant answers to the questions. She seemed to have it all just right, her answers were extremely spiritual and lofty and were filled with Scripture passages. However, it came to our attention that though she was married she was emotionally dependant upon another man–a married man, and they were planning a life together after divorcing their spouses.

"The one who says, 'I have come to know Him,' and does not keep His commandments, is a liar, and the truth is not in him" (1 John 2:4).

Sin first deceives and then it enslaves. Our objective at **The Lord's Table** Ministries is not just to help people lose a few pounds; it is to help them turn from all sin and learn to find satisfaction and contentment in Jesus. We desire to have people deal with the underlying issues they are using food to mask. It is important that our lives evidence the reality of our faith; that there is no area of sin to which we are in bondage (not that we don't sin, just that we should not be enslaved to habitual sin).

'The one who says he abides in Him ought to walk in the same manner as He walked.' That about says it all, doesn't it?

May we be enabled to forsake all deception, embrace the truth as it is in Jesus, and then convey this truth and reality to our students as well. This is all greatly honoring to the Lord, who came to set captives free from self-deception, from sinful bondage, and from all hypocrisy.

Challenge the class to examine their hearts and lives, and see if there is any sin cherished in the heart, and whether or not their lives evidence "keeping His commands" or do they just have "head knowledge."

Day 36

Question 1. Psalm 23:1 states "The Lord is my Shepherd". Is this true for you? If it is, then is the second phrase of the verse "I shall not want" (or lack) true also?

> Teachers: Help the class to see here that it is the leading of the Lord to green pastures (where He nourishes our souls), and quiet waters (where we peacefully drink of living water) that make us "not want." Our Great Shepherd meets our needs so that we do not have to wander away from the flock to seek satisfaction apart from the Shepherd.

Question 2. According to 2 Peter 1:3-4, what has God granted us?

> According to 2 Peter 1:3-4, God has granted us "all we need for life and godliness." This could mean that we have all needs provided for physically (life) and spiritually (godliness). One thing is for sure, we have no lack when we are seeking first the kingdom of God, He provides us with all that we need.

Day 37

Question 3. Romans 6:16-18 teaches that we were once slaves to sin, but are now slaves to righteousness. What does it mean to be a slave to righteousness, specifically as applied to the area of weight loss, eating right, exercise, etc.?

> Slaves are those who have no "free will" of their own to do as they please, but they are to only do their Master's bidding. We are those who have been freed from sin's control and rule in our lives by God's grace and now we are under the control and rule of righteousness, and as slaves of righteousness we eat in a disciplined manner at every meal, we exercise daily and we maintain self-control and moderation in all things.

Question 4. In 1 Corinthians 6:11, what three things may we expect God's Holy Spirit to do in our lives when we call on the name of the Lord Jesus?

> According to 1 Corinthians 6:11 when we become Christ's we are "washed," "sanctified" and "justified." This means that our natures

are completely changed and we receive new hearts with new passions and desires. We still have flesh that we war against, but the Holy Spirit undertakes the task of cleansing us from sin ("you were washed"), setting us apart from sin ("you were sanctified"), and declaring us righteous through Christ's shed blood on the cross ("you were justified").

This applies to us who, though we may have been Christians, have struggled fiercely with our weight. We must see the work of the Holy Spirit here as applying to this area of our lives, too. God's work is thorough and He makes us new in Him, and this includes the areas of our eating, exercise and discipline.

Day 38

Question 5. According to James 1:22, what is the only correct response to God's Word?

>According to James 1:22 the only correct response to God's Word is to be an "effectual doer" of the Word and not a "deceived hearer."

Teachers: At this point it would help to explain the difference between one who does the Word and will of God, and one who merely hears and so deceives himself.

A good example is the lady who went through nearly 50 days of **The Lord's Table** course, answering the questions correctly, providing much spiritual wordage in her answers, continually telling us how spiritual she was and how she used to teach God's Word, all the while she, as a married woman, was involved in a heart adulteress relationship with a married man. She was a "mere hearer" of the Word and she was deceiving herself. A "mere hearer" knows some Scriptures, maybe a lot of Scriptures, but because of lack of repentance and a clinging to idols he or she is merely hearing the Word of God, not effectually doing it.

A biblical example is the story Jesus told of two people who built houses; one built on a rock, the other built on the sand. When the rains and wind came the house on the sand fell flat while the house built on the Rock stood firm. Then Jesus tells us exactly how to build our lives on the Rock:

"Therefore everyone who hears these words of Mine and acts on them, may be compared to a wise man who built his house on the rock" (Matthew 7:24).

He also tells us how to build on sand: **"Everyone who hears these words of Mine and does not act on them, will be like a foolish man who built his house on the sand" (Matthew 7:26).**

Notice that both people heard the word of God, but only one "acted on" those words and obeyed them while the other merely heard the words but "did not act on them." There are many who read the words of Scripture, fewer will apply, obey, submit to and act on those words.

Question 6. Read Philippians 3:7-14. What is gained when we pursue Christ? What is the goal of pressing on?

> The goal of pressing on and pursuing Christ is to know Him. It is the enjoyment of relationship with Almighty God through His Son Jesus Christ that calls us to forsake sin and pursue Christ. The intimacy we experience with Christ enables us to leave behind all habitual sin.
>
> This passage states that Paul counted his entire past, all his religious training, his entire former life as "rubbish" so that he might know Christ. This insatiable desire to know Christ is a strong motivator for purity of life and overcoming sin.

Day 39

Question 7. How does Zephaniah 3:17-19 show us the way to victory?

> This passage shows us that victory is in Christ. When Christ is "in our midst" (verse 17) He "saves us" (verse 19) and turns our "shame into fame" (verse 19). This verse relates the centrality of Jesus Christ and the victory of His people. When Christ is central in our lives victory is sure.

Teachers: Help the students understand that victory does not come from sheer willpower but from Christ's power. Help them understand the futility of gritting our teeth and white-knuckling it to victory, instead our victory comes from Jesus Christ being "in the midst" of our lives. If we will focus on Him, count everything else loss (including diets, gimmicks, pills, programs) compared to knowing Him, seek Him first, He Himself will undertake for us and deliver us from habitual sin.

Day 40

Question 8. How does Luke 17:33 fit in with the idea of our being called to suffer and to die to ourselves?

> Luke 17:33 says, **"Whoever seeks to keep his life will lose it, and whoever loses his life will preserve it."**
>
> This statement by Jesus teaches us the necessity to let go of our life of self-gratification, to "die" to that entire way of living, that we might enjoy life abundant and eternal.

Jesus' statement follows the previous verse, "Remember Lot's wife" whom Jesus uses as an illustration of one who would not let go of her old life, so she lost her life. She "looked back" in longing for the pleasures and gratification that Sodom was known for, rather than "dying" to that old way of life and living in her new life of freedom from fleshy indulgence.

Help the students to make the connection, as Jesus did, between Lot's wife looking back with longing for the old life and our own life of self-gratification. Are we looking back and longing to gratify our cravings or are we dying to self-gratification and living in freedom from that "Sodom" lifestyle. The way to freedom is to die to the pleadings of the flesh (and we are referring here to OVEReating, not eating normal meals), to die to our entire past learning that the diet craze industry taught us, to die to all earthly wisdom, and to live in the enjoyment of relationship with Christ.

8:05-8:15 pm:
Final Teaching and Challenge: Living the Truth - Defined

"But the wisdom from above is first pure, then peaceable, gentle, reasonable, full of mercy and good fruits, unwavering, without hypocrisy. And the seed whose fruit is righteousness is sown in peace by those who make peace" (James 3:17-18).

The wisdom of God is defined by all the above traits, one of which is "without hypocrisy." This is the same as "living the truth" in 1 John 2:3-6 that we studied earlier. It is a characteristic of those who are living in wisdom that they have no deceit or guile, they do not pretend, nor do they have any areas of darkness that they frequent which must be concealed or hidden from others.

Instruct the class that sin, like a fungus, thrives in darkness and that the way to be free from it is to drag it into the light. Sin exposed becomes sapped of strength and it begins to wither and eventually die.

The teacher may want to share a personal testimony here of any time in his or her life that there was habitual sin and mask wearing, and how the grace of God enabled their freedom. This testimony can be followed by a general invitation to any who may be sinning in secret and wearing a mask to stay afterwards and discuss any issues that may be troubling them.

If any students do stay afterwards the teacher will want to look for idols of the heart, areas of deception, and help the student to turn from them, calling upon the Lord for forgiveness and freedom from sin.

Hand out questions for next week's lesson. Close in prayer.

Handout Questions for Group Discussion
Week 10

Day 41
Question 1. 1 Peter 2:21-24 begins, "**for you have been called for this purpose...**" What is the purpose?

Question 2. Read 1 Timothy 4:1-4. List the warnings in these verses. List what god has given us, and how we are to receive them.

Day 42
Question 3. Compare Proverbs 21:21 and Matthew 6:33. Give an example of something you want to change in the coming week so that you can fulfill Matthew 6:33 in your own life.

Day 43
Question 4. Consider Luke 10-38-42 again. Where did Jesus meet with Mary? Where was Mary's gaze?

Day 44
Question 5. According to 1 Corinthians 1:26-29, what qualifications are necessary for ministry?

Question 6. What gives us love for the brethren, and what kind of love will it be? (1 Peter 1:22,23).

Day 45
Question 7. Share one idea God brought to your mind as a vision for ministry.

Week Ten

7:00-7:05:
Call to Order and Opening Prayer

7:05-7:25:
Teaching: Idolatry of the Heart (1 Corinthians 10:7-14).

7:25-7:30:
Small break and reorganize into small group.

7:30-7:55:
Small Group Interaction

7:55-8:05:
Coming back together, singing two to three songs

8:05-8:15:
Teaching and Challenge - Illustration of Victory over Idols (1 Samuel 5:1-5)

Idolatry of the Heart

"**7Do not be idolaters, as some of them were; as it is written, 'THE PEOPLE SAT EAT AND DRINK, AND STOOD UP TO PLAY.' 8 Nor let us act immorally, as some of them did, and twenty-three thousand fell in one day. 9 Nor let us try the Lord, as some of them did, and were destroyed by the serpents. 10 Nor grumble, as some of them did, and were destroyed by the destroyer. 11 Now these things happened to them as an example, and they were written for our instruction, upon whom the ends of the ages have come. 12 Therefore let him who thinks he stands take heed that he does not fall. 13 No temptation has overtaken you but such as is common to man; and God is faithful, who will not allow you to be tempted beyond what you are able, but with the temptation will provide the way of escape also, so that you will be able to endure it. 14 Therefore, my beloved, flee from idolatry" (1Corinthians 10:7-14).**

This passage teaches the truth that "God is a jealous God" (Exodus 20:5) and shows us the horrible effects of idolatry. Idolatry is defined here as those who "ate and drank, and rose up to play" and worship the golden calf. This event happened while Moses was receiving the law on Mt. Sinai and it was when the people built a golden calf for themselves to worship, having turned away from the Living God. This is the definition of idolatry: anything that turns our hearts away from worshiping God.

Idolatry happened when the Israelites were gluttonous drunkards (1 Corinthians 10:7) and they turned from the worship of God to the golden calf they had made. Idolatry for us happens when our thoughts become consumed with something other than God, when our hearts long for something other than Jesus, when our desires are so strong for something that we will sin in order to get it.

Notice in the 1 Corinthians 10 passage that four specific things are mentioned in the condemnation of the Israelites, and let us examine our own hearts as we read through this list (note to teacher - pause after noting each item on the list below, giving the students time to reflect):

- Eating and drinking (in a manner of gluttony and drunkenness), verse 7
- Playing. This is not the healthy kind of "playing" that would characterize normal recreation or sports activity, but rather the "revelry" that is mentioned in Exodus 20, the kind of "partying" that throws restraint to the wind and is characterized by indulgence, verse 7.
- Immorality, verse 8.
- Trying or testing the Lord, verse 9.
- Grumbling, verse 10.

These sins committed by the Israelites, and the subsequent displeasure and wrath of God, are recorded in this passage as an "example" to us, and for our "instruction" (verse 11). We are to "learn" from these events and take heed to the warning presented to us, which warning is written at the end of this passage, "therefore my beloved, flee from idolatry" (verse 14). Yes, this is the lesson we are to learn, get away from idolatry as fast as possible.

The human heart was designed to worship. It MUST worship something or someone. When the heart finds something other than God to worship, it is idolatry. We want the Spirit of God to shine the light of truth into the hearts of students present, to see if there is anything they might be clinging to that is hindering real worship of the living God through His Son Jesus Christ.

Day 41

Question 1. 1 Peter 2:21-24 begins **"for you have been called for this purpose. . ."** What is the purpose?

> The purpose for which we were called is to suffer. The context of this passage makes it clear that this suffering is for doing right. When we are harshly treated for doing right we find favor with God if we bear up under it, just as Jesus was falsely accused and reviled, yet He did not revile back but bore up under the suffering.

> Even though the context of 1 Peter 2 instructs us that we were called to suffer for doing right, yet the cross of Jesus Christ is not limited to this. Jesus also suffered physically because He refused to bypass the cross. Because He chose the cross, He not only suffered in His soul as He bore the sin-weight of all believers, but He also suffered in His body.

> In some sense, we are called to this type of suffering as well. If we choose to crucify our flesh instead of gratify it there will be inevitable suffering. We were called to this suffering when Jesus said, **"And he who does not take his cross and follow after Me is not worthy of Me" (Matthew 10:38).**

Question 2. Read 1 Timothy 4:1-5. List the warnings in these verses. List what God has given us, and how we are to receive them.

> The warnings are about listening to and following those who are deceived, who teach things contrary to God's Word, such as the forbidding of marriage and the denial of certain foods.

> According to this passage we are to receive "all things" with thankfulness, and reject nothing. This passage is not an excuse to indulge in all kinds of things, but rather to receive all things with

thanksgiving. We cannot receive something that we are indulging our flesh in with thanksgiving, so this passage does not call us to indulgence but rather to acceptance of all foods with thankfulness.

It is so important to apply this teaching to the diet craze industry, that attempts to foist on the public a denial of certain foods. Each body is made up differently and we are instinctively given the ability to discern which foods are not good for our particular system. Some, being lactose intolerant, should not eat dairy foods, others need lots of milk because of the good calcium it provides, whereas others profit from a diet high in meat products, and so on. Each person is unique.

Day 42

Question 3. Compare Proverbs 21:21 and Matthew 6:33. Give an example of something that you want to change in the coming week so that you can fulfill Matthew 6:33 in your own life.

Day 43

Question 4. Consider Luke 10:38-42 again. Where did Jesus meet with Mary? Where was Mary's gaze?

> Jesus met with Mary as she sat at His feet and listened to His Word. This is the posture of submission, of learning, of worship. Mary is a good illustration of Matthew 6:33, knowing that if she sought Jesus first that all other things would be taken care of. Jesus commends this understanding and encourages Mary that she is doing the "one thing needful."

To apply this teaching to our subject of weight loss, far more would be accomplished by seeking Jesus first than to count calories, fat grams, or make sure we had the exact amount of each of the "required" food items. If we seek to humble ourselves as Mary, who sat at Jesus' feet, if we seek a relationship with Jesus ahead of everything else, if we seek to worship God as our primary activity, we will be more successful than if we followed the exact recommendations of a diet guru.

This "success" is because our hearts are changed in the presence of God, our "appetites" (loves, desires, etc.) are affected by being in God's presence, and our motives are purified. God makes sure that "all things" are added unto us if we seek Him first and there is lasting change that happens when we are in God's presence. **"Now the Lord is the Spirit, and where the Spirit of the Lord is, there is liberty. But we all, with unveiled face, beholding as in a mirror the glory of the Lord, are being transformed into the same image from glory to glory, just as from the Lord, the Spirit" (2 Corinthians 3:17-18).**

Day 44

Question 5. According to 1 Corinthians 1:26-29, what qualifications are necessary for ministry?

> God chooses the "weak, foolish, miserable and despised" to use in ministry, for He is honored greatly when He doesn't have much to work with. God does not choose the best of the best to lead and minister, He chooses the lowly, the humble, the foolish. All of us at one time or another have been weak, and some of us have been foolish, which leads to being miserable and despised. Our weakness can be used to help others to strength, and our foolishness can make others wise, and God gets all the glory.

Question 6. What gives us love for the brethren, and what kind of love will it be? 1 Peter 1:22,23?

> Purity precedes passion. Purity of heart enables us to love each other fervently (from the heart). When we, by purifying our souls, love each other from the heart, we become the greatest evangelistic tool the church has. We who have overeaten, but are now seeking purity in Christ by ridding our lives of habitual sin, will find that our love for the brethren results in many ministry opportunities.
>
> The greatest hindrance to true ministry is impurity. When we set out, by God's grace, to purify our hearts, we become clean vessels, useful to the Lord.

"Now in a large house there are not only gold and silver vessels, but also vessels of wood and of earthenware, and some to honor and some to dishonor. Therefore, if anyone cleanses himself from these things, he will be a vessel for honor, sanctified, useful to the Master, prepared for every good work. Now flee from youthful lusts and pursue righteousness, faith, love and peace, with those who call on the Lord from a pure heart" (2 Timothy 2:20-22).

Setting Captives Free was founded because of God granting purity of heart and life to a couple who then desired to love others the way that Christ was loving them and setting them free from habitual sin.

Day 45

Question 7. Share one idea God brought to your mind as a vision for ministry.

Read Luke 8:26-56. Who were the three people healed by Jesus from these verses? Each of them had a different problem - what was it? Once healed, how did each one respond to Jesus?

This question is designed for discussion.

8:05-8:15 pm:
Final Teaching and Challenge: Living the Truth—Defined

"Now the Philistines took the ark of God and brought it from Ebenezer to Ashdod. Then the Philistines took the ark of God and brought it to the house of Dagon and set it by Dagon. When the Ashdodites arose early the next morning, behold, Dagon had fallen on his face to the ground before the ark of the LORD. So they took Dagon and set him in his place again. But when they arose early the next morning, behold, Dagon had fallen on his face to the ground before the ark of the LORD. And the head of Dagon and both the palms of his hands were cut off on the threshold; only the trunk of Dagon was left to him. Therefore neither the priests of Dagon nor all who enter Dagon's house tread on the threshold of Dagon in Ashdod to this day" (1 Samuel 5:1-5).

This passage of Scripture shows us the power of the presence of God to defeat idols. The ark of God had been captured by the Philistines and taken away from the people of God and placed in the house of the heathen god Dagon. It is instructive to read from Dr. Thomas D. Rodgers on this story:

> "Chapter 5 tells how the Ark of God was taken from the battle site over to Ashdod, which was one of the five Philistine cities by the Mediterranean seacoast. In true henotheistic fashion, they set up the Ark in the house of their god Dagon. To them, the Ark was the God of the Israelites and they would worship it also along with their fish-headed god Dagon.
>
> "But God demonstrated very dramatically that He was not just another idol. When the philistines entered their temple the next morning, they found that Dagon had fallen on his face. They set him up, but the next morning he had fallen on his face again. This time his head and the palms of his hands were cut off. The fish head idol was humiliated and mutilated in its own temple." [3]

The important truth to catch here is that it was the presence of God that knocked down the idol. God was demonstrating not only His superiority over any idol, but the manner in which to knock them down. Idols are knocked down by God's presence.

When we consider what it takes to truly overcome overeating and laziness we must conclude that only the presence of Almighty God can help. It is not enough to merely change our diet because we need more than that, we need a heart change and a lifestyle change. As we seek God first and seek to enthrone Him in every room of our body-temples, the idols will fall.

Hand out questions for next week's lesson. Close in prayer.

Handout Questions for Group Discussion
Week 11

Day 46

Question 1. Read 1 Peter 5:5. What can we expect from God if we are proud? What can we expect if we are humble?

Question 2. Psalm 145:14-21 gives us a picture of humility and worship. How do these heart attitudes maintain our freedom from overeating?

Day 47

Question 3. Read Galatians 5:22-23. Self-control is a result of what?

Question 4. How does abiding in Christ and He in us give us the proper perspective or focus?

Day 48

Question 5. Read Hebrews 9:22-28. How is Christ the "reality", the fulfillment of the law?

Question 6. In Hebrews 10:1, 10-14, what has Christ provided for us?

Day 49

Question 7. Read Mark 1:35. What was Jesus doing, and when?

Question 8. Read Psalm 19:14. Is there a correlation between the object of our mediation and our speech?

Day 50

Question 9. Read 1 Peter 1:2. What enables us to be obedient? What is the result of our obedience?

Question 10. How does Psalm 1 teach us to be doers of the Word?

Week Eleven

7:00-7:05:
Call to Order and Opening Prayer

7:05-7:25:
Teaching - The Purpose of Freedom: Praise (Psalm 30).

7:25-7:30:
Small break and reorganize into small groups

7:30-7:55:
Small Group Interaction

7:55-8:05:
Coming back together, singing two to three songs

8:05-8:15:
Teaching and Challenge - Illustration of The Power of Praise

The Purpose of Freedom: Praise

A Psalm of David: [1]I will extol You, O LORD, for You have lifted me up, and have not let my enemies rejoice over me. [2]O LORD my God, I cried to You for help, and You healed me. [3]O LORD, You have brought up my soul from Sheol; You have kept me alive, that I would not go down to the pit. [4]Sing praise to the LORD, you His godly ones, and give thanks to His holy name. [5]For His anger is but for a moment, His favor is for a lifetime. Weeping may last for the night, but a shout of joy comes in the morning. [6]Now as for me, I said in my prosperity, "I will never be moved.."[7]O LORD, by Your favor You have made my mountain to stand strong; You hid Your face, I was dismayed. [8]To You, O LORD, I called, and to the Lord I made supplication: [9]"What profit is there in my blood, if I go down to the pit? Will the dust praise You? Will it declare Your faithfulness? [10]Hear, O LORD, and be gracious to me; O LORD, be my helper."[11]You have turned for me my

mourning into dancing; You have loosed my sackcloth and girded me with gladness, that my soul may sing praise to You and not be silent. O LORD my God, I will give thanks to You forever" (Psalm 30).

This Psalm teaches us the method and the purpose of our freedom. The method is to call upon the Lord, and the purpose is that we might praise the Lord. David says, "I cried to You for help, and You healed me" (verse 2), "To You, O Lord, I called, and to the Lord I made supplication" (verse 8), and "Hear, O Lord, and be gracious to me; O Lord, be my Helper" (verse 10). So David "cried," "called" and "made supplication." We get the sense in this passage that David went often to the Lord for help, and that He approached God earnestly crying out for grace. This is the recipe for success in all of life. If we would beseech the Lord for help, crying to Him in earnestness and pleading for His grace, making sure we've repented of any known sin, God will hear us and help us as He did David.

When we are seeking to lose weight the most effective thing we can do is not to read up on the latest "healthy" foods, nor learn how many calories we must limit our diets to, or exactly how many fat grams are in the food we eat, but rather it is to come humbly to the Lord and ask Him for help, crying out to Him for grace. If we do this we, too, like David, will have the testimony "I cried to You for help, and You healed me" (verse 2). Our testimony should NOT be that we found freedom through any program, or diet, or pills, but rather that the Lord Himself heard our cry for help and He healed us.

But then what is the reason that God hears the prayer of sinners and heals them from their backsliding? It is so that they might live a life of praise, extolling the worth and faithfulness of God all the day long and into eternity.

David declared what God had done for him in verse 11, and in verse 12 he tells us the reason why with the word "that." In verse 11 David said that God had turned his mourning into dancing and had removed his sackcloth (symbol of repentance) and clothed him with gladness. In verse 12 he tells us why God did this in his life, "That my soul may sing praise to You and not be silent. O LORD my God, I will give thanks to You forever."

"That" is an important word. It explains the purpose of God's work in David's life, and in ours; THAT we might sing praise and give thanks eternally. You see, the work of God is to rescue us from the power of sin that we might praise Him eternally.

So now we understand the method of finding victory over sin as well as the purpose of our salvation. We are to cry out to the Lord in repentance, to plead for His grace, and when He delivers us we are to be about praising the Lord. When we turn our attention to the Lord like this, and focus on Him, both in seeking His grace for change and in praising Him for His answer, we live free from habitual sin and become testimonies of His amazing grace. Joining the "Jesus Watchers" program in this manner glorifies God and brings more victory into the life than joining a diet plan or weight loss program.

Day 46

Question 1. Read 1 Peter 5:5. What can we expect from God if we are proud? What can we expect if we are humble?

> God resists the proud. This literally means that He keeps them away from him, He "stiff-arms" them. God pushes proud people away from Him, not desiring their company. But if we humble ourselves God gives us grace, and grace is what is so needed to find victory over sin.

Question 2. Psalm 145:14-21 gives us a picture of humility and worship. How do these heart attitudes maintain our freedom from overeating?

> The Lord Himself "raises up all who are bowed down" with humility. Victory over sin comes from bowing down in humility before the Lord, humbling ourselves in His presence and then experiencing His grace that lifts us up to victory.

Day 47

Question 3. Read Galatians 5:22-23.   Self-control is a result of what?
Where does it originate? (hint: not self)

> Self control is a fruit of the Holy Spirit. It comes from God as
> the Holy Spirit indwells us. This is why it is absolutely critical to
> receive new birth from God in order to overcome sin in our life.
> Self-control is the result of the Holy Spirit living within us. Of
> course people can lose weight without the assistance of the Holy Spirit,
> but true self-control, the control over every area of life, is only
> given to those who are in Christ.

Question 4. How does abiding in Christ and He in us give us the proper
perspective or focus?

> This question is presented for discussion purposes.

Day 48

Question 5. Read Hebrews 9:22-28. How is Christ the "reality", the
fulfillment of the law?

> Jesus Christ is the substance or "reality" of all Old Testament laws and
> shadows. He is, for the believer, our "rule for life." He is both our
> Savior and our Lord, our Redeemer and our Example.

Question 6. In Hebrews 10:1, 10-14, what has Christ provided for us?

> Jesus Christ has provided both justification (declaring us not
> guilty of our sins) and sanctification (progressively enabling us to
> gain victory over our sins). This sanctification is a gift of grace,
> just as justification is, and it results in a life of discipline,
> self-control, and moderation; in other words, a life lived without
> excess in any area.

Day 49

Question 7. Read Mark 1:35. What was Jesus doing, and when?

> Jesus Christ was seeking His Father early in the morning. Just as the Israelites gathered fresh manna daily, and had to do so before the sun got hot, so Jesus was up gathering fresh grace from His Father early in the morning. He sought God in prayer in the first part of His day.

Question 8. Read Psalm 19:14. Is there a correlation between the object of our meditation and our speech?

> Out of the overflow of the heart, the mouth speaks. The Christian desires that both the thoughts and the words will be honoring to the Lord, so He often meditates upon the Lord and speaks of Him.

Day 50

Question 9. Read 1 Peter 1:2 What enables us to be obedient? What is the result of our obedience?

> Our obedience, according to this passage of Scripture is enabled by the sanctifying work of the Holy Spirit. It is God, the Holy Spirit, Who works in our hearts, giving us both the desire and the ability to obey Him.

Question 10. How does Psalm 1 teach us to be doers of the Word?

> Psalm 1 teaches us that it is only those who "do" the Word that will be fruitful. Those who do not walk in the counsel of the ungodly, those who do not stand in the way of sinners or sit in the seat of mockers, are blessed by God and made fruitful by God. Those who meditate on and delight in God's Word, for the purpose of doing it in obedience, are blessed with a fruitful life.

8:05-8:15 pm:
Final Teaching and Challenge: The Power of Praise – Illustrated

In the earlier session we discovered that the purpose of our salvation
is that we might live a life of praise to God. This praise comes from
our hearts as God releases us from bondage to sin and sets us free to
worship Him. But praise of God is also itself a very freeing experience,
for God "dwells in the praises of His people." This truth, that God
lives in the praises of His people, is illustrated very clearly in the
following story by Robert and Bobbie Wolgemuth. As we read this story,
and see the freeing power of praise, may our hearts be encouraged to
lift up worship to our Almighty God.

*"She probably won't recognize you," Dr. James Dobson said to Bobbie and
me as he ushered us into his aging mother's hospital room. "Yesterday
she didn't know who I was."*

*In a few minutes we were sitting on the edge of Myrtle Dobson's bed.
Suffering from Parkinson's disease, which rendered her confused, she was
unable to speak more than a word or two at a time. At first we didn't
know if she recognized anyone in the room, but she was awake and seemed
alert. Dr. Dobson spoke kindly to his mother, graciously reminding her
who we were, even though we had known her very well. She nodded and
smiled.*

*After a few minutes of small talk, Bobbie spoke up, "Why don't we sing.
Myrtle loves to sing."*

> *O worship the King all-glorious above,*
> *O gratefully sing His pow'r and His love;*
> *Our shield and Defender, the Ancient of Days,*
> *Pavilioned in splendor and girded with praise.*

*For the first few lines of the hymn, she silently smiled back at us.
Could she understand? Was she listening? We really couldn't tell.*

*As we sang a final verse, Myrtle's eyes began to sparkle. We knew she
recognized this great hymn. Her mouth began first to form the words;*

then she joined in with each unforgettable word. What was even more amazing than Myrtle's remembering the lyrics to this great hymn was the fact that she sang a perfect alto. Many hymns followed, and she almost flawlessly recalled nearly every word.

The music may not have been strong enough to land a record contract, but it was good enough to fill our hearts with enough gratitude and praise to last a lifetime.

> Frail children of dust, and feeble as frail,
> In you do we trust, nor find you to fail,
> Your mercies how tender, how firm to the end,
> Our Maker, Defender, Redeemer and Friend

Dr. Dobson wept almost uncontrollably at the familiar sound of his mother singing this great melody of faith.

That afternoon we got a glimpse of the fullness of God's complete and perfect grace. This once vigorous woman, no longer having the capacity to even stand, was the picture of "frail children. and feeble as frail." But as the faithful wife of an artist, college professor, and traveling evangelist, her heart sang of God's trustworthiness. And as the mother of an active and gifted son, she knew of God's inability to fail.

Now, at the close of her life Myrtle Dobson was singing of God's tender mercy, good to the very end.

This hymn includes what may be the most powerful four-word summary of the character of the Sovereign God of the Universe ever recorded: "Maker, Defender, Redeemer, and Friend." Think of it! Maker: He created us. Defender: The forces of evil melt at the sound of His name. Redeemer: The death of His own Son was not too high a ransom to pay. Friend: A woman too weak to sit without help had Someone who reassured her of His everlasting presence.

As we drove away from the small hospital that Sunday afternoon, a light rain began to fall. For the first few minutes there was no talking, only the rhythmic sound of the windshield wipers. What we had experienced was too holy, too sanctified to discuss.

Almost two years later Myrtle Dobson went home to be with her Lord. Some of the well-wishers at the visitation reminded Dr. Dobson of his mother's great love of life and wonderful humor. Years before she had quipped that she thought her tombstone should read, "I told you I was sick!" They all laughed as they remembered.

But no one needed to be reminded that this precious woman had finished well. At an early age she had been introduced to the King as her personal Savior and had spent her life being filled with awe and worshiping Him. And now she could sing in His very presence in exquisite harmony.(Used by permission). [4]

Hand out questions for the next week's lesson. Close in prayer.

Handout Questions for Group Discussion
Week 12

Day 51

Question 1. How does Galatians 2:20 fit in with overcoming gluttony and laziness?

Question 2. What can we learn from the ant in Proverbs 6:6-11?

Question 3. In John 4:16-18 and John 8:11, Jesus clearly confronts sin, but without condemnation. Why is it vital to confront sin?

Day 52

Question 4. Read Romans 12:1-2. How do we present our bodies as a living and holy sacrifice? How do we renew our minds?

Question 5. Consider 2 Corinthians 10:5 again. What does it mean to "take every thought captive to the obedience of Christ"?

Day 53

Question 6. From reading Psalm 27:8 and Psalm 105:4, what are we to seek? How often?

Day 54

Question 7. What do you see in Isaiah 40:11 as to how God shepherds His sheep?

Day 55

Question 8. The Lord Jesus Himself shared many meals with the apostles and others. On the eve before His death He broke bread and ate with them. What was His purpose? (Matthew 26:20, 26-29).

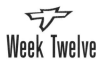

Week Twelve

7:00-7:05:
Call to Order and Opening Prayer

7:05-7:25:
Teaching: Who's In Control? (The Sovereignty of God).

7:25-7:30:
Small break and reorganize into small groups

7:30-7:55:
Small Group Interaction

7:55-8:05:
Coming back together, singing two to three songs

8:05-8:15:
Teaching and Challenge: The Sovereignty of God - Illustrated

Who's In control?
(The Sovereignty of God)!

As we near the end of **The Lord's Table** course there will most certainly have been much heart work that the Lord has done and is doing in those who have persevered with the study. This is because God uses His Word to reach into the heart of those who seek Him, and He make changes that are often quite astounding to both the people with whom He is working, and others around them.

Some of the changes God makes in hearts, through His Word, will bring up many questions by the students. Some of these questions are: Will I surrender my need for control and recognize His? Will I give up my life dreams and allow Him to be my one consuming passion? If I do, will He be enough? What about when I'm faced with losing a loved one? Is He able to sustain me when my whole life falls apart? Will I know beyond a doubt that He still loves me and will carry me through the deep valleys?

For others, it is still about weight loss, as well. If I have a LOT to lose, can I stick with it for the long haul?

It is impossible to cover all the questions that can arise when God is at work in the hearts of His people. There are simply too many issues that He roots out and that people need help in dealing with.

But let us take this brief time together to seek the Lord for answers to the sample questions raised above, and we will see that understanding the sovereignty of God is the answer. God's Word has the answer, and as teachers we must seek to help others apply His Word in their own lives as they deal with their own unique circumstances. So let's look to God's Word.

Overeating has often been the symptom of the deeper problem of "control." Those who seek to "control" things in their lives, and especially those who use food as a means of control (whether they overeat, or starve, binge and purge) are often lacking the biblical understanding of the Sovereignty of God. While they might give mental assent to the simple statement, "God is in control of all things" their practical outworking of this truth in their lives, their desire to control and be in charge of certain areas, show that they don't really believe or understand it fully. The one who struggles with being a "control freak" needs to truly grasp the sovereignty of God, as stated in the following passages:

"But at the end of that period, I, Nebuchadnezzar, raised my eyes toward heaven and my reason returned to me, and I blessed the Most High and praised and honored Him who lives forever; for His dominion is an everlasting dominion, and His kingdom endures from generation to generation. All the inhabitants of the earth are accounted as nothing, but He does according to His will in the host of heaven and among the inhabitants of earth; and no one can ward off His hand or say to Him, 'What have You done?'"(Daniel 4:34-5).

King Nebuchadnezzar lived in pride and ruled his kingdom as if he were in control of it all, until God humbled him by sending him out to pasture where he temporarily lost his sanity for a period of seven years. At the end of that time Nebuchadnezzar learned some valuable lessons about the sovereign control of God. He said, God "does according to His will in the host of heaven and among the inhabitants of earth."

Nebuchadnezzar came to understand that God is in control of all things, that He does as He pleases with all people, and that He is sovereignly in control of every event that happens, whether it seems good or bad.

Now this truth that God is sovereign does not deny man's responsibility. Earlier God gave Nebuchadnezzar one full year to repent of his pride as he was responsible to do after God confronted him with it. Yet Nebuchadnezzar refused to repent and God held him accountable for his failure and chastised him in what might appear to be a very severe way. God was in control, but Nebuchadnezzar was responsible.

The truths of God's sovereignty and man's responsibility are not at odds with each other but are both true and are both taught in Scripture.

The one who struggles with "control" needs to learn to bow to the sovereignty of God, just as Nebuchadnezzar had to learn the truth and bow to it as well. God is in control at all times, with all people, and in every event.

[9]"He made known to us the mystery of His will, according to His kind intention which He purposed in Him [10] with a view to an administration suitable to the fullness of the times, that is, the summing up of all things in Christ, things in the heavens and things on the earth. [11] In Him also we have obtained an inheritance, having been predestined according to His purpose who works all things after the counsel of His will" (Ephesians 1:9-11).

This passage might seem somewhat wordy at first glance, but it is important to grasp the truth of it so that we can see the sovereignty of God. Verse 11 is the focus of the passage, showing that God "works all things after the counsel of His will." The "all things" that God is working according to the counsel of His own will are inclusive of every event, every detail of life, everything that happens to each person. He is the sovereign Ruler and Lord of all of life.

Sometimes it is difficult for people to grasp this concept because they know the devil is alive and well and that he wreaks havoc among people, and they know that people have the capability of choosing between several options. How can God be in control when the devil does so much damage and when people have the capability of making their own decisions and choices?

The answer is that God is at work behind every event and every decision made. When speaking of the evil that is done in the world, prompted by the devil and carried out by evil people, it is important to understand that God is in control of that as well. Let's take just one example, the worst evil ever committed by man, the crucifixion of Jesus Christ. We note that evil men committed this act, **"For truly in this city there were gathered together against Your holy servant Jesus, whom You anointed, both Herod and Pontius Pilate, along with the Gentiles and the peoples of Israel" (Acts 4:27).**

Yes, evil men gathered together against Jesus and they did those evil deeds that was in their hearts to do, crucifying the Lord Jesus Christ. They are also responsible for their actions and will be held accountable for them, as other Scriptures make clear.

But why did they do those things? Why did they crucify the Lord of glory? The next verse in Acts tells us why. Let's read the passage in context:

27"For truly in this city there were gathered together against Your holy servant Jesus, whom You anointed, both Herod and Pontius Pilate, along with the Gentiles and the peoples of Israel, 28 to do whatever Your hand and Your purpose predestined to occur" (Acts 4:27-8).

We note in verse 28 that the evil men gathered against Jesus and crucified Him because they were doing "whatever Your hand and Your purpose predestined to occur." That's right, God predestined the crucifixion of His Son. He planned and purposed it, and was in control of it all. He predestined the death of His Son Jesus so that all who believe would be saved, and He was in control of all the details it took to bring it about.

Those who seek to "take control of their lives" must learn the truth that God is in control and that He does not surrender His sovereignty to anyone at any time. Though we are responsible for our actions, accountable for our choices, and though all will be called into account for the lives they have lived, ultimately God is in control and "works all things according to the counsel of His own will." This is important to those desiring control be-cause it is freeing! It helps us to know that we do not need to assume control of our lives because God is already in control. He is sovereign over all details of our lives, and He is working out all things in our lives according to the counsel of His own will.

Now some will say that this teaching makes us all robots, or puppets on a string. This is untrue. We are humans, we have reasoning capabilities, we have intelligence, we have the ability to make decisions based upon logical input. However, behind it all, God is working. He is at work in the big plans of our lives and in the little details. He is in control of our going and our coming, our choices and decisions, our attitudes and actions. Yes, we are responsible for our decisions and actions, but God is in control.

Proverbs 16:9 is an important verse that helps us with these truths. It says, **"The mind of man plans his way, but the LORD directs his steps."** This tells us we are not robots for we have "minds" that are able to make "plans" and determine which "way" to go. However, behind it all is a loving God Who "directs our steps." We make our plans, but the Lord directs our steps. He is in control. He is sovereign over which way we go.

Finally, when dealing with this issue of "control" and the sovereignty of God, some would be tempted to accuse God of evil doing, which can never be true. They might say, "Well, if God is in control of everything, then He could have prevented my father's cancer, or the loss of my job, or even my own condition of being overweight." While that statement is true, the fact that God did not prevent these things does not make Him evil. God is good, all the time. God plans, purposes, and predestines all things for good. This is important. Notice a couple of verses:

And we know that God causes all things to work together for good to those who love God, to those who are called according to His purpose. For those whom He foreknew, He also predestined to become conformed to the image of His Son, so that He would be the firstborn among many brethren (Romans 8:28-9).

This passage tells us that God causes all things to work together for good to those who love Him and are called according to His purpose. If you are a Christian who loves God, who has been called to Him for fellowship and intimacy, He is "behind the scenes" of your life causing all things to work together for good. He is able to take the "bad" things that happen to us, and even our own sin, and cause it all to work together for His glory and our good. He is able to take what the devil means for evil and bring good out of it. God is sovereign, and God is good. All the time. In everything. Understand it, believe it, trust it. And then relinquish your own desires for control, recognizing that God is already in control. Bow to His sovereignty and His loving rule in your life, and find freedom from trying to take control yourself.

We need to surrender our own self-will, surrender our lives in their entirety, to the sovereign control of God. He bought us, He owns us, He loves us, He is in control.

Day 51

Question 1. How does Galatians 2:20 fit in with overcoming gluttony and laziness?

> In Galatians 2:20 Paul states the truth that he is dead with Christ and that the life he now lives he lives by faith in Christ. As Christians we died with Christ to gluttony and laziness, and the life we live is the life of resurrection power to overcome these sins. Dead people can't sin.

Question 2. What can we learn from the ant in Proverbs 6:6-11?

> The ant is compared to the sluggard in this passage. The ant is busy at work, preparing for the future, whereas the sluggard is lazy and becomes impoverished. We are to learn from the ant the importance of hard work, of diligence, of preparing for the future. We are to learn from the ant not to be lazy, not to be a sluggard.

Question 3. In John 4:16-18 and John 8:11, Jesus clearly confronts sin, but without condemnation. Why is it vital to confront sin?

> Biblical confrontation is the means God uses to affect change in the heart and life of a believer. The world denies or seeks to "support" someone who is sinning whereas believers are to love the person who is sinning enough to lovingly confront them. Jesus did. We should too.

Day 52

Question 4. Read Romans 12:1-2. How do we present our bodies as a living and holy sacrifice? How do we renew our minds?

> This question is for discussion and personal input from the students.

Question 5. Consider 2 Corinthians 10:5 again. What does it mean to "take every thought captive to the obedience of Christ"?

> Within this verse many truths are taught. One of the main ones is that the mind is a battlefield. The evil one can place thoughts in our minds that are unholy, our own flesh manufactures thoughts that are ungodly, and the world bombards us with words and pictures that are profane. We are not to allow these thoughts to rule over us but instead we are to take these thoughts captive to Christ.

Day 53

Question 6. From Psalm 27:8 and Psalm 105:4, what are we to seek? How often?

> These verses describe the life of a Christian, who is to be about seeking the face of God continually. There are many distractions to this life of continually seeking God's face, and many of us have become distracted by the lifestyle of laziness and gluttony, which have a disastrous effect on our spiritual life. As we turn away from these twin sins we discover that our spiritual life is renewed so that we have divine energy to seek the face of God and being in His presence.

Day 54

Question 7. What do you see in Isaiah 40:11 as to how God shepherds His sheep?

> Isaiah 40:11 says, **"Like a shepherd He will tend His flock, in His arm He will gather the lambs and carry them in His bosom; He will gently lead the nursing ewes."**

This picture of God as a Shepherd describes His work among His people in four ways:

> He tends
> He gathers

He carries
He leads His people.

He "tends" His flock, which is another way of saying that He pastures and grazes His flock, or that He rules His flock, and even that He associates with His flock. All of these terms are contained within the Hebrew word to "tend."

He "gathers" His flock, which means that He grasps, collects and assembles His flock.

He "carries" His flock next to His heart. This shows His tender and loving compassion for His people. Those who are tired are carried by God.

He "leads" His flock. He goes before us. One preacher said, "God is already into Thursday" meaning that when we arrive at Thursday God has already been there so whatever happens to us has been filtered through and ordained by Him. He goes ahead of us, He leads us, we follow Him.

Day 55

Question 7. The Lord Jesus Himself shared many meals with the apostles and others. On the eve before His death He broke bread and ate with them. What was His purpose? (Matthew 26:20, 26-29).

> Jesus ate the "last supper" with His disciples and used the food as symbols of His death, fellowshiping with them in the meaning of that death. He said the bread was His "body" and then He broke it and gave it to the disciples who then ate it, He then poured the wine and gave it to the disciples who drank it, indicating that we are to "feed" on and be "nourished" by His death and the blood He shed for the forgiveness of our sins.

It is intended that we fellowship with Jesus Christ around food. Food, and especially **The Lord's Table**, is to remind us of our communion with God because of the death of His Son. We have spiritual and eternal life because Jesus died, and food is to be a continual reminder of the price Jesus paid in order that we receive the nourishment of His death for us.

Practically, whenever we eat we should meditate on the Lord, on the blessing we have in Christ, and we should "assimilate" these benefits to our soul just as our bodies assimilate the food.

8:05-8:15 pm:
Final Teaching and Challenge: The Sovereignty of God—Illustrated

The life of Joseph provides us with an amazing account of one who was mistreated, abused, neglected and falsely accused. Yet in all his trials, Joseph knew the hand of God was upon Him and he trusted in the sovereignty of God, knowing that God was working all things for his good.

Joseph was sold by his brothers to some Ishmaelite traders who then sold him into slavery in Egypt. He was industrious and trustworthy and so was promoted to the house of Potiphar and became ruler over the household. But then he was falsely accused by Potiphar's wife and thrown into prison where he remained for 3 years. Finally he was released and brought up from prison to become Pharaoh's right hand man, leading the nation of Egypt through good times and bad, and providing food for all the surrounding nations.

When Joseph's brothers came to him for food during a famine, and when Joseph revealed his identity to them, they became exceedingly afraid of what Joseph might do to them in retaliation for the wrongs they did to him. But Joseph understood the sovereignty of God; that God was in control of all things. That understanding enabled him to respond in a way that honored God. When the brothers were afraid of being punished for their wrongs Joseph said,

"Do not be afraid, for am I in God's place? As for you, you meant evil against me, but God meant it for good in order to bring about this present result, to preserve many people alive" (Genesis 50:20).

Joseph knew that the brothers meant evil to Joseph in selling him into slavery, but He also knew that God meant it for good. God was behind it all, working out His purpose in it all, controlling all events and details that it took to get Joseph to Egypt.

The one who understands the sovereignty of God is able to respond to the cruelty of others in a manner that honors the Lord.

And finally, it is of tremendous interest to see that the sovereignty of God in the life of Joseph was working out all things to be a picture of Jesus Christ, that we might grow in faith, having further evidence to believe in Him. Consider these details in the life of Joseph and how they point forward to our blessed Lord Jesus Christ:

Joseph was loved by his father but hated by his brothers. His father sent Joseph on a mission of mercy to check on his brothers, but when they saw him coming they plotted his death. They sold him into the hands of Gentiles for pieces of silver. He was falsely accused and thrown into prison where he was numbered with the transgressors. He was placed right between two criminals to whom he brought a message of life to one and a message of death to the other. He was then released from his tomb-like prison and exalted to the right hand of Pharaoh where he became ruler over all and the savior of the known world, providing bread to all who came to him.

Yes, God is in control. He worked out all the details of the life of Joseph, He works out all details of our lives as well. We can trust Him. He means us good. He means to bring glory to Himself and good to us through everything that happens in our lives.

Though there will be some who mean to do us evil in our lives, behind them is a God who uses their acts for good to bring us blessing instead of curses. God is in charge; He is on the throne ruling all events, taking all that the devil does to us and all that evil people do, and even our own sin, and using it for good in our lives.

No, this does not give us an excuse to sin as if to say, "Oh, God uses even sin for His glory and our good, I guess I will sin in order to bring Him more glory and myself more good." No, that is foolish and blasphemous, and indicates a heart that is not subdued by God's grace.

The sovereignty of God is not to be used as a means to allow us to sin. The sovereignty of God is to show us how God uses all things, including sin, to accomplish His purposes. The sovereignty of God is to encourage us that His plans and His purposes can never be thwarted and that He will do all His good pleasure in our lives, completing the work He began, so as to bring Himself the maximum amount of glory and us the maximum amount of good.

Job learned this lesson, and so should we: **"I know that You can do all things, and that no purpose of Yours can be thwarted"** (Job 42:2). God's purposes cannot be thwarted. This is good to know. This is freeing to know. God is in control. He will accomplish His plans and purposes to do us good. Of this we can be sure.

Hand out question sheets for next week's lesson. Close in prayer.

Handout Questions for Group Discussion
Week 13

Day 56

Question 1. According to Psalm 95:6-7, what is the appropriate response to our God?

Day 57

Question 2. Read 1 Peter 1:21,22. What is the outcome of being purified through obedience to the word of God?

Day 58

Question 3. Instead of talking/complaining about weight loss, we are given the privilege to sing praises to God as He sets us free. What do you read that encourages you in Psalm 146:1,2, 8-10 and 147:1-6?

Day 59

Question 4. Please share specific verses and/or biblical principles from the course that impacted you and that the Holy Spirit used to change you and set you free.

Day 60

Question 5. Please share a brief testimony to God's grace in your life over the last three months.

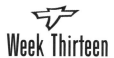

Week Thirteen

As we bring these meetings to a close, we want to leave the class understanding that for the child of God victory is guaranteed, it is inevitable, it is assured.

Karen Wilkinson is a **Setting Captives Free** board member, Mentor Coordinator and secretary to Mike Cleveland, and she writes,

"There is no question of whether we will have victory from habitual sin, because that has already been taken care of on the cross. The war has been won, as well as all the battles. It is not about us and our strength or weakness, but about Him and His strength. Because of our position in Christ, we have resurrection power. He has overcome and we are now overcomers with him, not overeaters."

It is important to understand that defeat in the life of the Christian is temporary. Times of self-indulgence are transitory and they give way to a life of victory in Jesus Christ that is permanent.

No, we never reach perfection in this life, we need to continually strive for the mastery, continually press toward the mark of the high calling of Christ, and to be vigilant against temptation and sin. Yet Jesus' promise that we would be not just free from sin's power but "free indeed" should resonate within our hearts and minds as we look at living our remaining days. The main mission of the Messiah is to set captives free. Victory is assured.

Today, we are going to share our testimonies and provide some feedback on the course, but before we do we want to spend a few minutes examining the connection between quenching our thirst in Jesus Christ and overcoming sin with all of its deception. Victory in Jesus is inevitable for the believer, but it is not automatic. It requires diligence in pursuing the face of God, purposefully neglecting other things in order to seek Him, and daily quenching our thirst in Him. We're not referring here to neglecting important things that must be done, but rather extraneous things that can indeed be neglected without negative consequences to the life.

Note the following passage briefly:

"'5And He who sits on the throne said, 'Behold, I am making all things new.' And He said, 'Write, for these words are faithful and true.' 6Then He said to me, 'It is done. I am the Alpha and the Omega, the beginning and the end. I will give to the one who thirsts from the spring of the water of life without cost. 7He who overcomes will inherit these things, and I will be his God and he will be My son. 8But for the cowardly and unbelieving and abominable and murderers and immoral persons and sorcerers and idolaters and all liars, their part will be in the lake that burns with fire and brimstone, which is the second death'" (Revelation 21:5-8).

This passage is worth a long period of meditation for there is much to stir the passion for God and to rouse us to heart devotion. God is shown here as the One who:

- Makes all things new - verse 5
- Freely quenches the thirst of His people - verse 6
- Shares a special relationship with those who overcome - verse 7
- Punishes those who refuse to repent - verse 8

It is highly instructive to note the order of verses 6 and 7. Please look at them again: In verse 6 God promises to give living water to the thirsty and in verse 6 He promises blessings to those who overcome. Please note that quenching of thirst precedes overcoming. Did you catch that? Those who learn to drink from Jesus, those who become skilled at satisfying their hearts in Christ, are those who overcome sin and experience the blessing of God. This is ever the order of Scripture, and the sure means to victory.

Yes, victory is assured for God's people. In fact it is because Jesus died to provide it and therefore it is certain for all believers. And yet it is not automatic or involuntary, rather it is achieved by those who learn to drink in Jesus and satisfy their souls in Him.

As this course draws to a close, please challenge the students to go and drink of Christ; to go and quench their thirst in Him; to go and satisfy their heart and soul in Him. Help them to understand that it is not enough to be disciplined in eating or to maintain daily accountability, for the thirst of the soul must be quenched in order to truly overcome and to receive God's blessing.

Close this teaching session by reading the following Scriptures, noting the victory that is ours in Christ:

"Jesus answered them, 'Truly, truly, I say to you, everyone who commits sin is the slave of sin. The slave does not remain in the house forever; the son does remain forever. So if the Son makes you free, you will be free indeed" (John 8:34-36).

"These things I have spoken to you, so that in Me you may have peace. In the world you have tribulation, but take courage; I have overcome the world" (John 16:33).

"The sting of death is sin, and the power of sin is the law; but thanks be to God, who gives us the victory through our Lord Jesus Christ. Therefore, my beloved brethren, be steadfast, immovable, always abounding in the work of the Lord, knowing that your toil is not in vain in the Lord" (1 Corinthians 15:56-58).

"I am writing to you, little children, because your sins have been forgiven you for His name's sake. I am writing to you, fathers, because you know Him who has been from the beginning. I am writing to you, young men, because you have overcome the evil one. I have written to you, children, because you know the Father. I have written to you, fathers, because you know Him who has been from the beginning. I have written to you, young men, because you are strong, and the word of God abides in you, and you have overcome the evil one" (1 John 2:12-14).

"You are from God, little children, and have overcome them; because greater is He who is in you than he who is in the world" (1 John 4:4).

"For whatever is born of God overcomes the world; and this is the victory that has overcome the world—our faith. Who is the one who overcomes the world, but he who believes that Jesus is the Son of God?" (1 John 5:4-5).

Day 56

Question 1. According to Psalm 95:6-7, what is the appropriate response to our God?

> Psalm 95:6-7 make it clear that worship is the appropriate response to God. We kneel before the Lord for He is our maker, we worship Him for He is our Redeemer. As God redeems us from bondage to overeating and laziness the appropriate response is one of whole-hearted worship.

Day 57

Question 2. Read 1 Peter 1:21,22. What is the outcome of being purified through obedience to the word of God?

> Love is the outcome of purity. We cannot truly love others while we are indulging our own flesh and living a lifestyle of self-gratification. 1 Peter 1:22 tells us that purity precedes passion, godly passion, as we are enabled to love others fervently when our hearts are purified by grace.

Day 58

Question 3. Instead of talking/complaining about weight loss, we are given the privilege to sing praises to God as He sets us free. What do you read that encourages you in Psalm 146:1,2, 8-10 and 147:1-6?

> This question is designed to solicit discussion and interaction among the students.

Day 59

Question 4. Please share specific verses and/or biblical principles from the course that impacted you and that the Holy Spirit used to change you and set you free.

Day 60

Please share a brief testimony to God's grace in your life over the last three months.

The Lord's Table Leader's Guide

Appendix

Appendix A
The Believer and the Flesh

Christians often wonder why they sin. If it is true that we are "new creations in Christ," then why do we feel weak against temptation and seem at times to be powerless to resist? Why do Christians sin?

A partial answer to this is that Christians have "flesh" which is weak (Matthew 26:41), and of course the devil, who is strong as a roaring lion. What is this "flesh" and how are we to gain victory over it?

Some have used the term "sinful nature" instead of "flesh," but this is not an accurate concept biblically for the believer, and it leads to a false identity for the struggling Christian. Christians do not have a "sinful nature," rather; we have "flesh." The difference is one of definition and identification. Let's explain this a little further:

People of the world who have not become converted, or born-again (John 3:3-5), have a sinful nature. As we are born into this world in sin, we have a nature that is sinful (Psalm 51:5). This nature which loves to do sin continues until conversion, at which time it is put to death and we are given a new nature. This is salvation, which is a radical transformation in our inner being.

At salvation we are not merely granted a new nature, while retaining our old nature. That would be addition. Salvation is not addition but rather transformation. In salvation the "old man" is put to death and our new man is born, thus "we" are born again.

So Christians are "new creations in Christ." Their old nature, or "old man" was nailed to the cross with Christ and he lives no more. In practical terms, salvation brings about a radical change in the heart, in the mind, will and emotions; indeed in the very nature of the new creature.

Some, when reading the above material, would become quite discouraged if we put an end to it there. It seems to leave no room for Christians who sin, or worse yet, for those who become temporarily trapped in sin. They could become overly discouraged and think that since they don't seem to evidence a totally new nature, or their heart and passions are at times divided, they might not be truly converted.

But the above discussion is not complete, and we must add an additional thought from Scripture. The truth is that Christians not only have a new nature, (the old one having been crucified with Christ), but that new nature lives in flesh and the flesh is that which trips up believers.

The flesh is the "residue" of the old man, or "that which remains of wickedness" (James 1:21). It is described as "weak" (Matthew 26:41) and "at war" with the Spirit of God (Galatians 5:17). We are instructed to "crucify" it and the crucifixion of the flesh is shown to be the mark of a true Christian (Galatians 5:24).

So, Christians sin because they have flesh that they have not learned to crucify daily, and they are allowing it to lead them. While our inner man, which is our true self (our real identity), longs to do what is right, the flesh at times can prevent him from doing so. As believers grow in grace their new man becomes stronger and gains the weapons necessary to deal forcefully and effectively with their flesh on a daily basis.

For **The Lord's Table** study it is not essential to communicate these truths about the flesh, the new nature, etc., but it is important to understand them and be able to help those who ask.

Endnotes

1. Henry, Matthew, *Matthew Henry's Commentary on the Whole Bible: Complete & Unabridged*, Peabody, MA, Hendrickson Publishers, 1991.

2. Bunyan, John, *Pilgrim's Progress*, Ulrichsville, OH, Barbour & Co., 1985.

3. Rodgers, Thomas R., *The Panorama of the Old Testament*, pg. 126, Trinity Press, 1998.

4. Wolgemuth, Robert and Bobbie, Tada, Joni Eareckson, MacArthur, John, *O Worship the King* - Hymns of *Assurance and Praise to Encourage Your Heart*, pp. 33-35, Crossway Books, Wheaton, Ill.

Notes